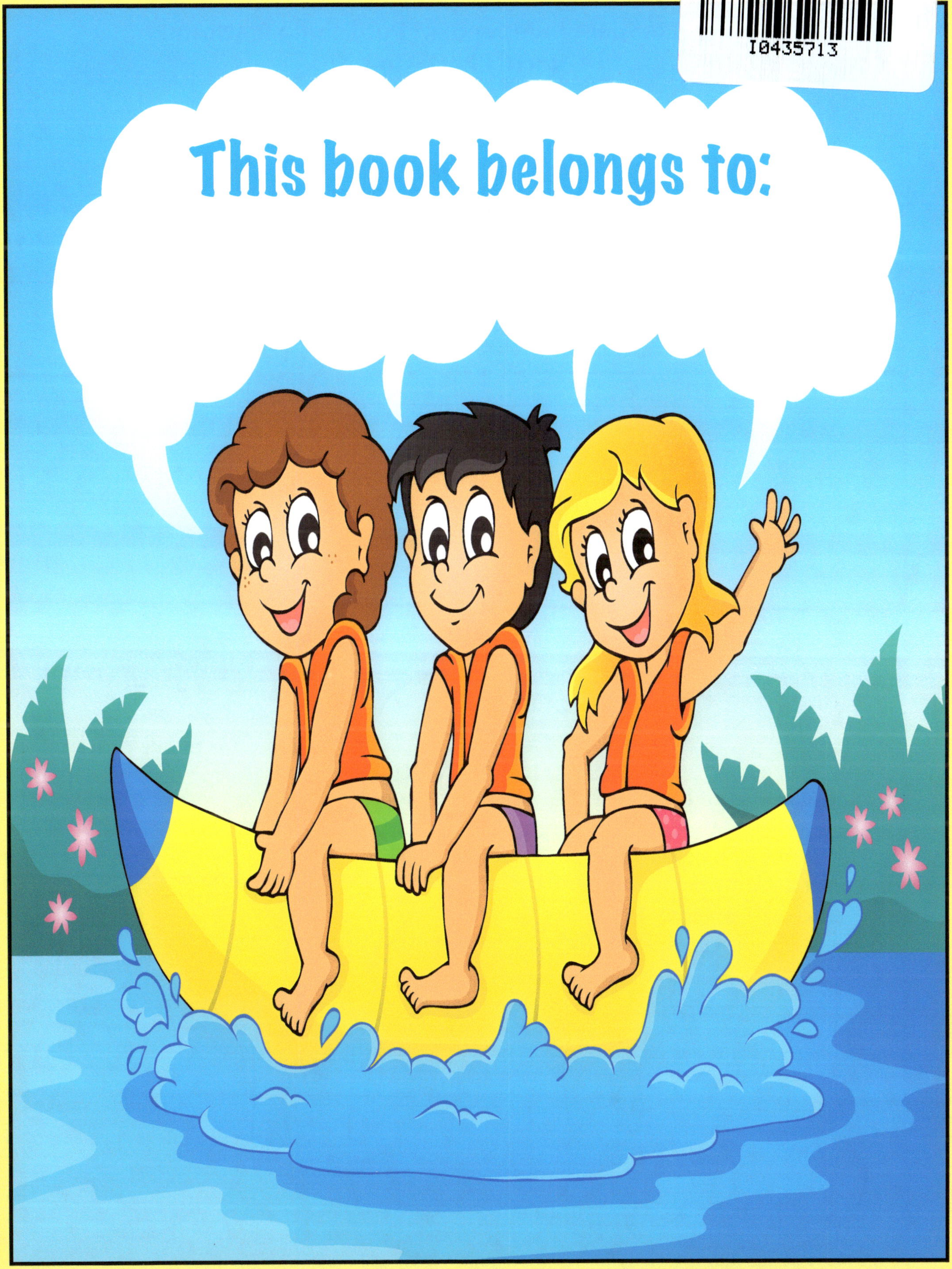

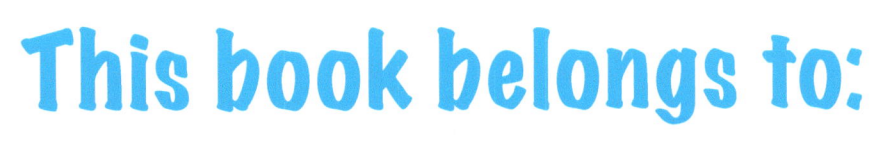

This book belongs to:

Library of Congress Control Number: 2016904190
CreateSpace Independent Publishing Platform
North Charleston, SC

Copyright ©2016 Mary Lou Brown & Sandy Mahony

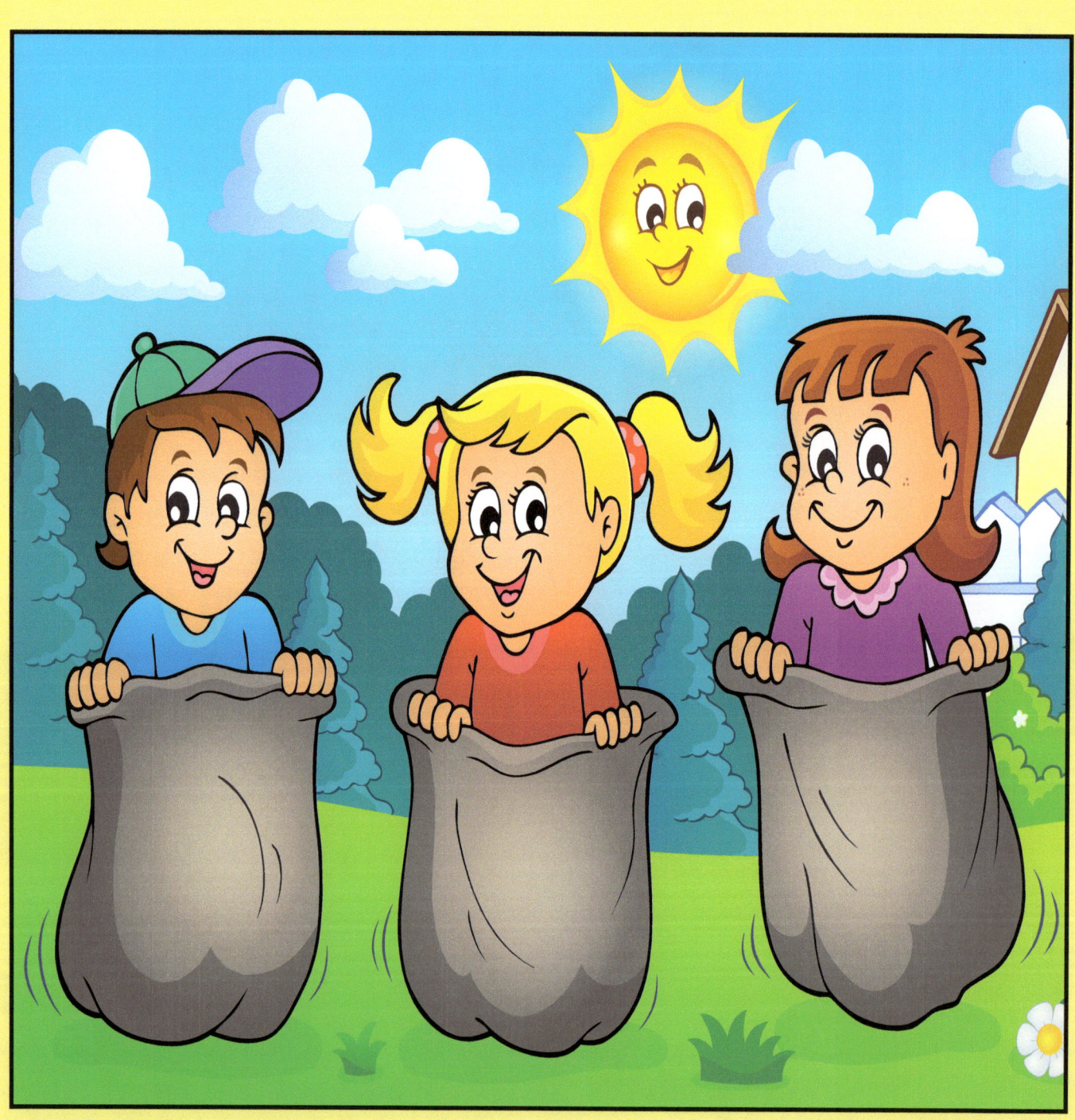

Fit Kids Have Fun!

Mary Lou Brown & Sandy Mahony

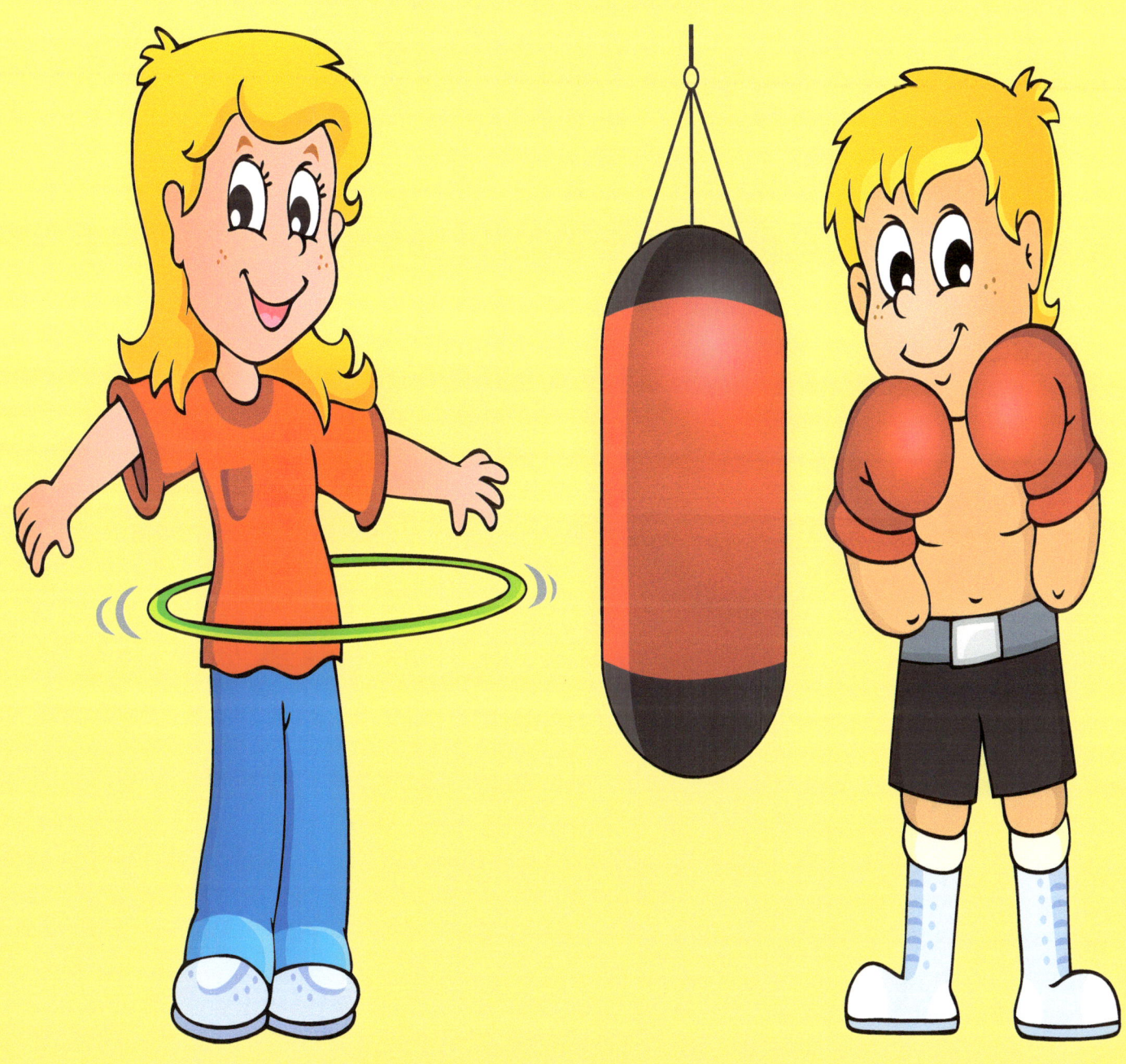

An Alphabet Book of Active Play

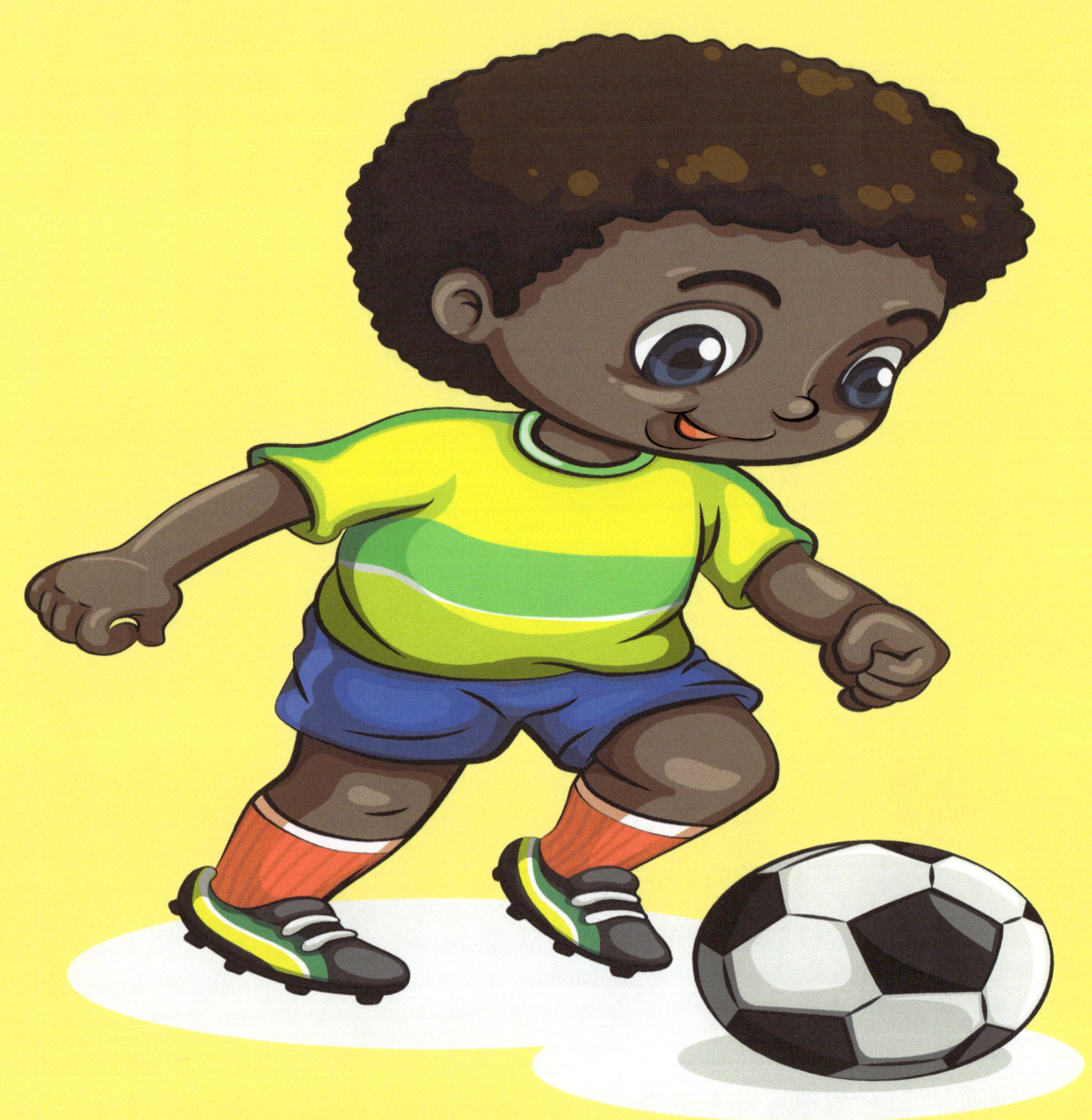

Hi everyone, Jackson here.
Lively friends will soon appear.
Active kids are fun and fit.
Moving, playing, they won't quit!
Action words I often use.
About each sport they give clues.
The alphabet will show the way,
sixty minutes of play each day!

Archery

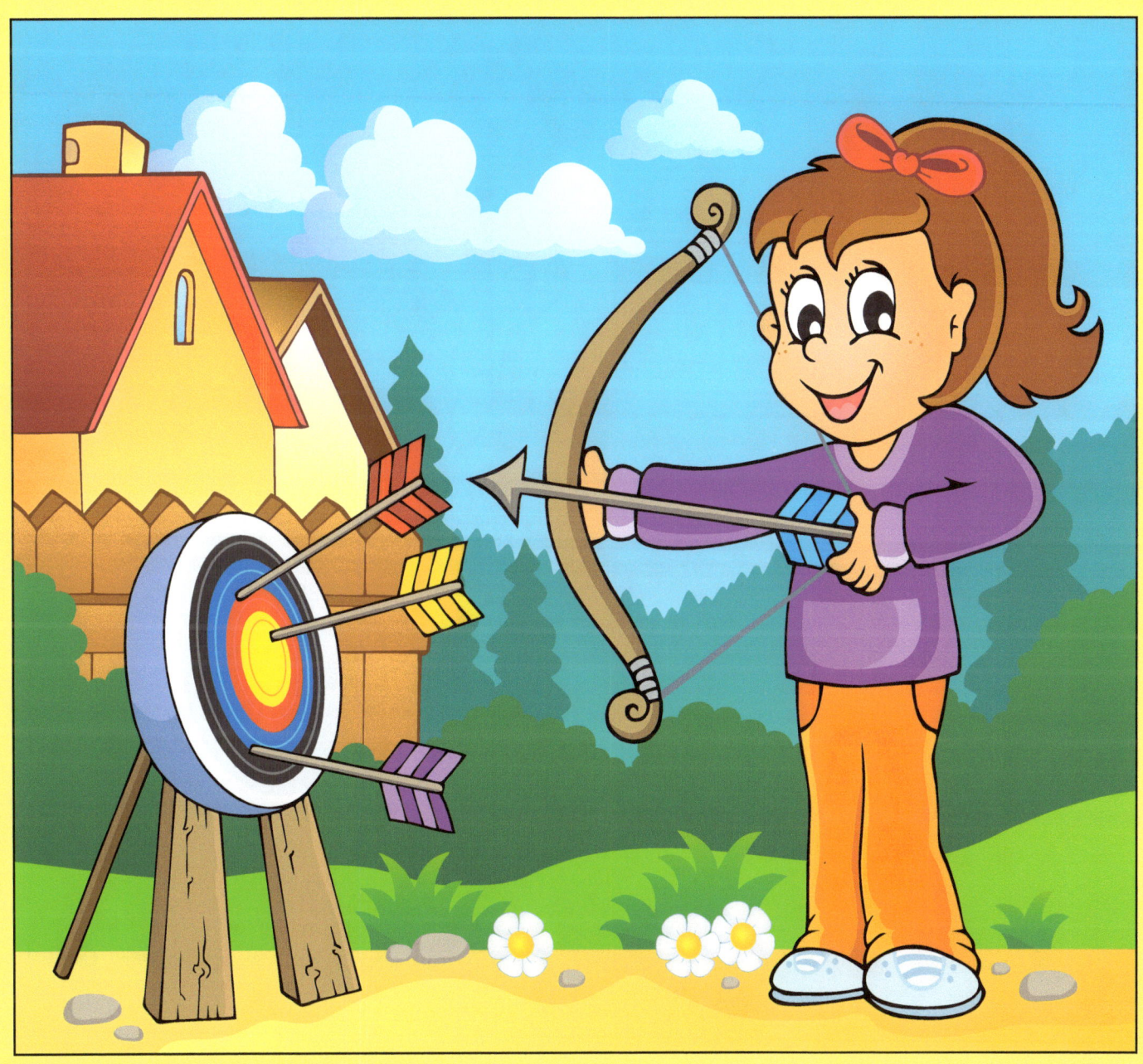

Shooting the arrow from the bow,
straight to the target it will go.
Take aim and let the arrow fly,
fast and sure toward the bullseye.

Basketball

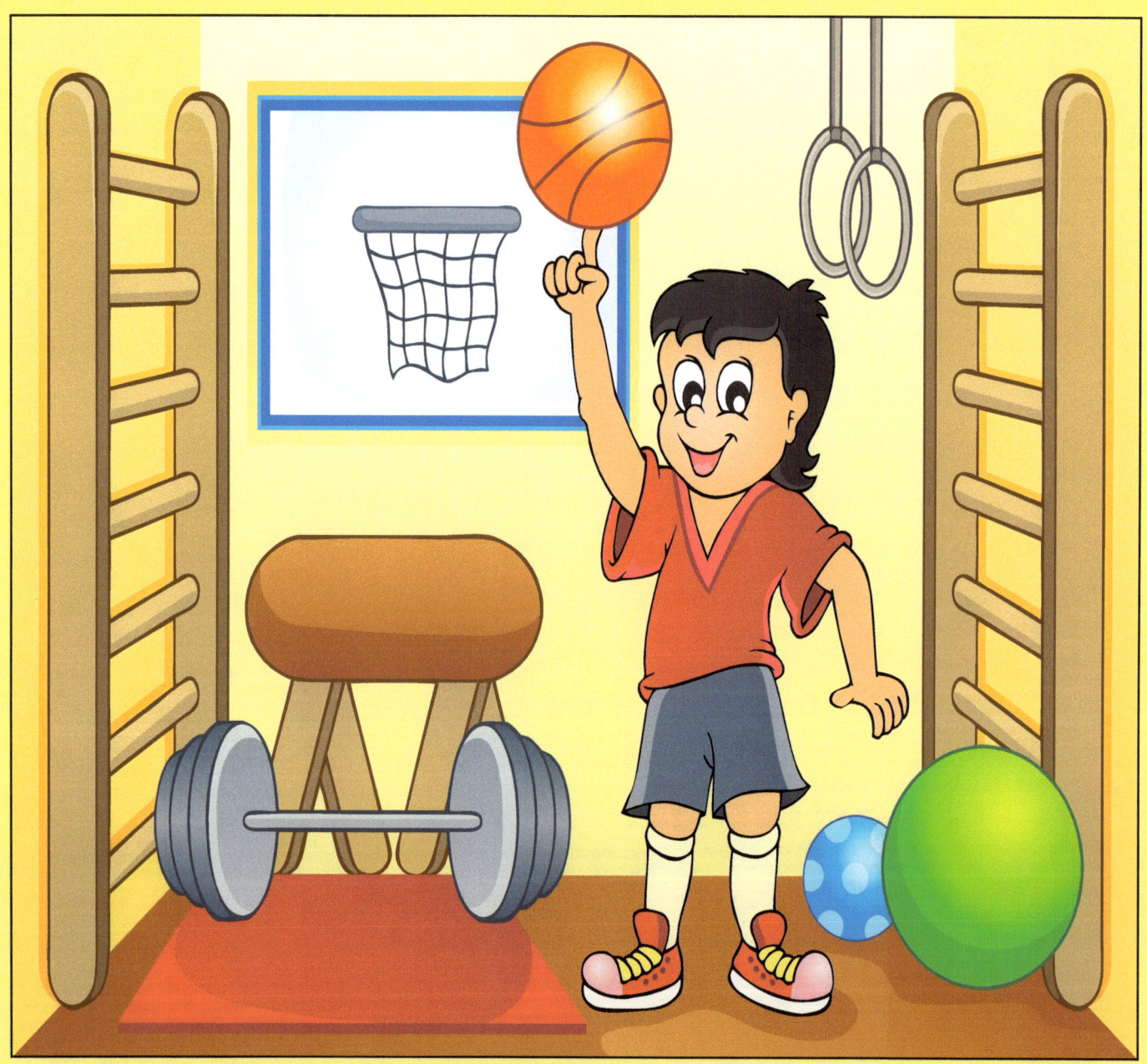

I dribble the ball down the court.
Basketball is a fast team sport.
Two or three points I will get,
pass, shoot, and swish through the net.

Climb

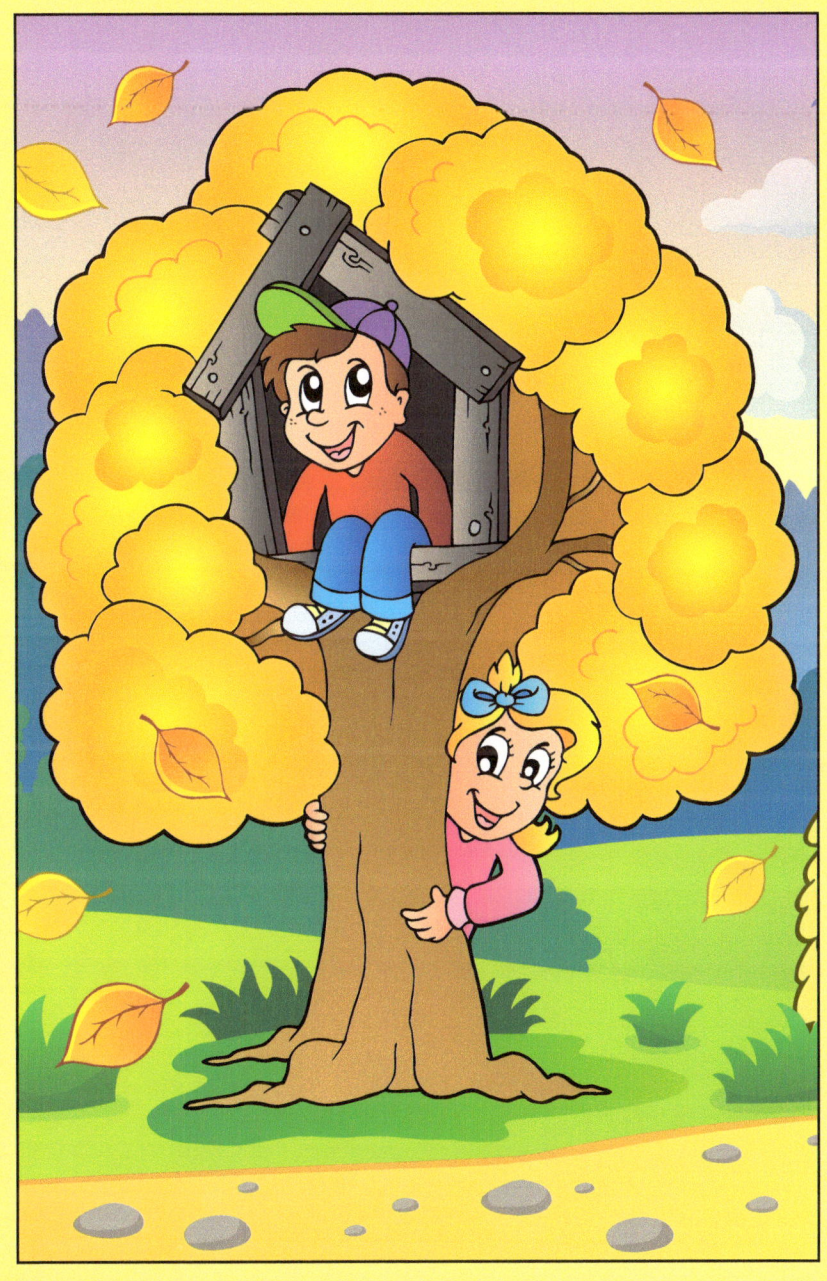

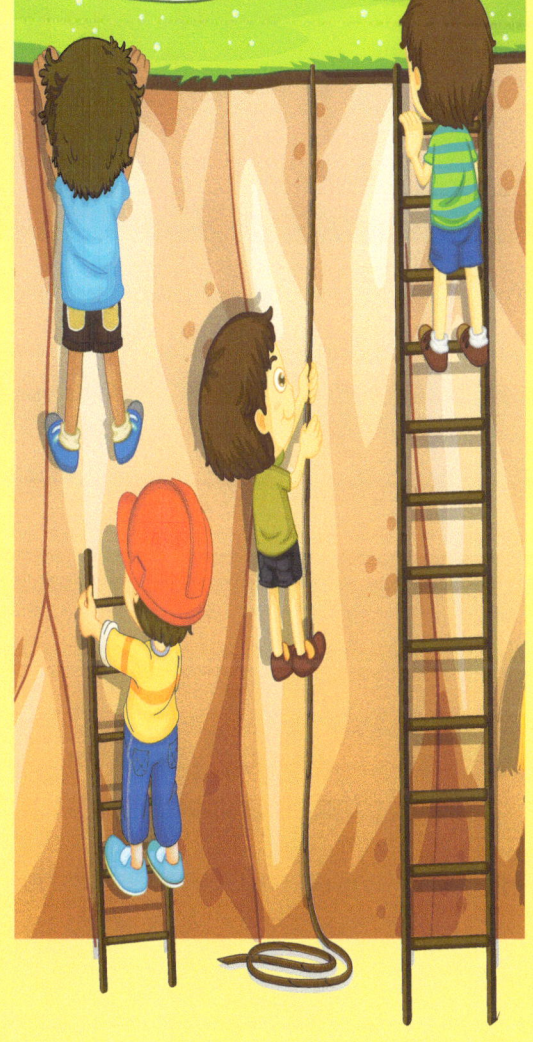

A tree, tall mountain,
ladder, or hill;
I carefully climb.
Oh, what a thrill!

Dodgeball

Ducking, dodging, don't get hit by the ball!
Dodgeball, a quick sport, I don't want to fall.
Hurl the ball at the other team.
Hit someone and they're out is the theme.

Exercise Bike

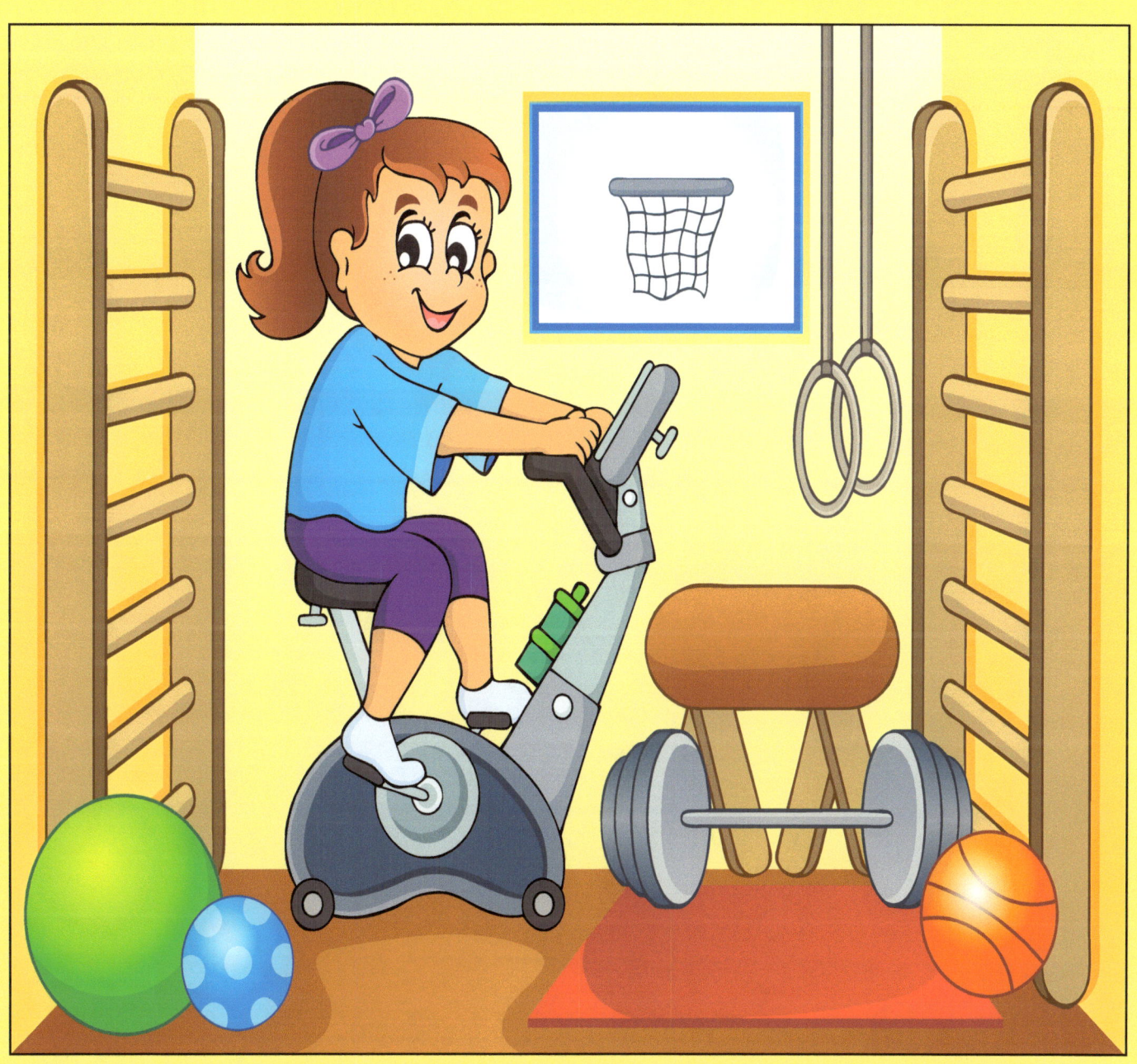

Riding an exercise bike is easy to master.
I get a better workout if I pedal faster,
I don't need a gold or silver medal.
I just need to pedal, pedal, pedal!

Fly a Kite

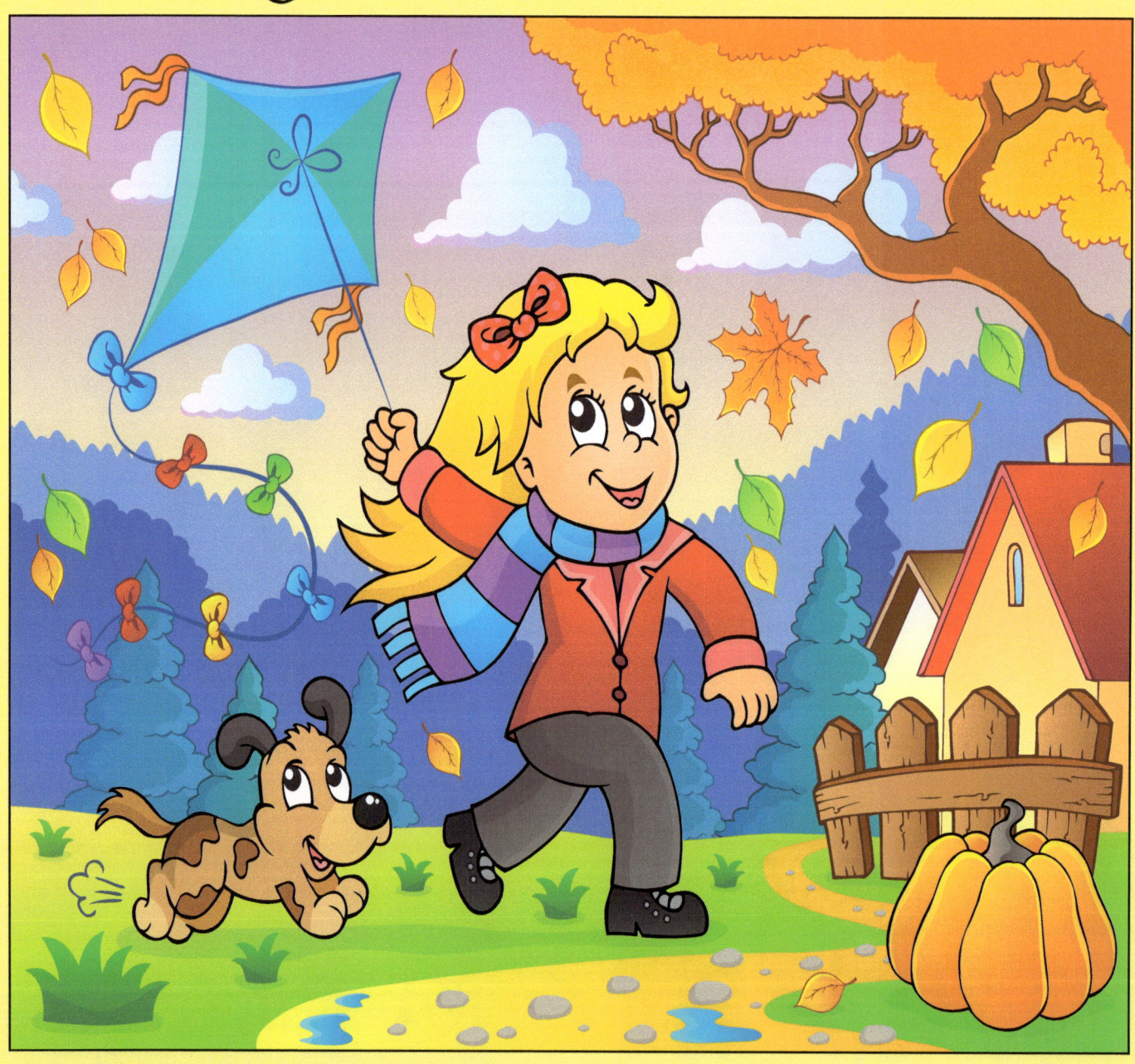

I hold the string very tight,
running and flying my kite.
The wind makes it dip, dive, and fly,
way up high in the cloudy sky!

Golf

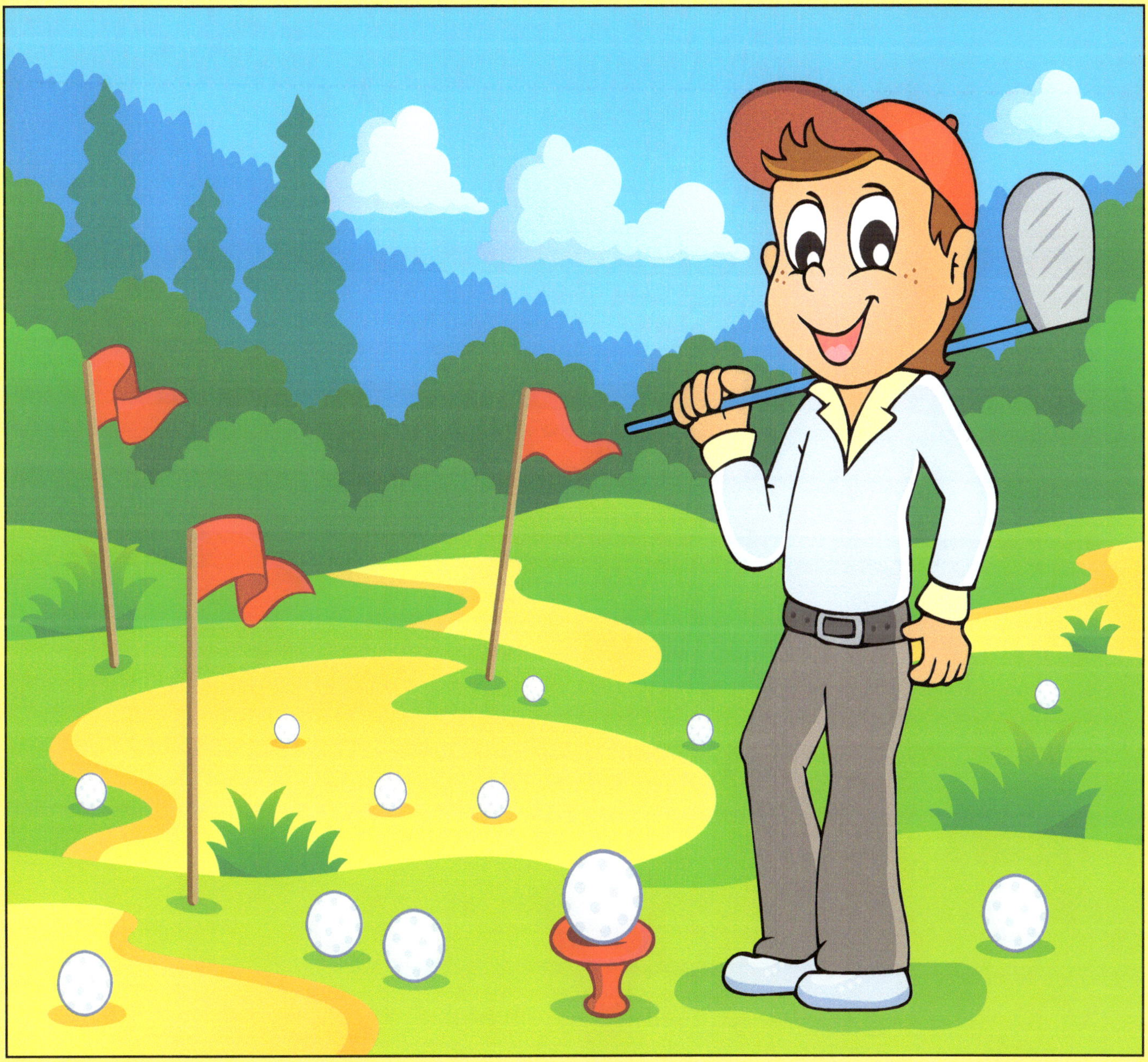

Swinging the club, driving the ball,
hoping, in the hole it will fall.
Add all strokes, each hole more,
golfers want a low score.

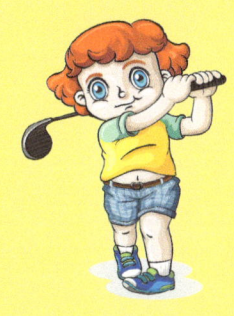

Hop Scotch

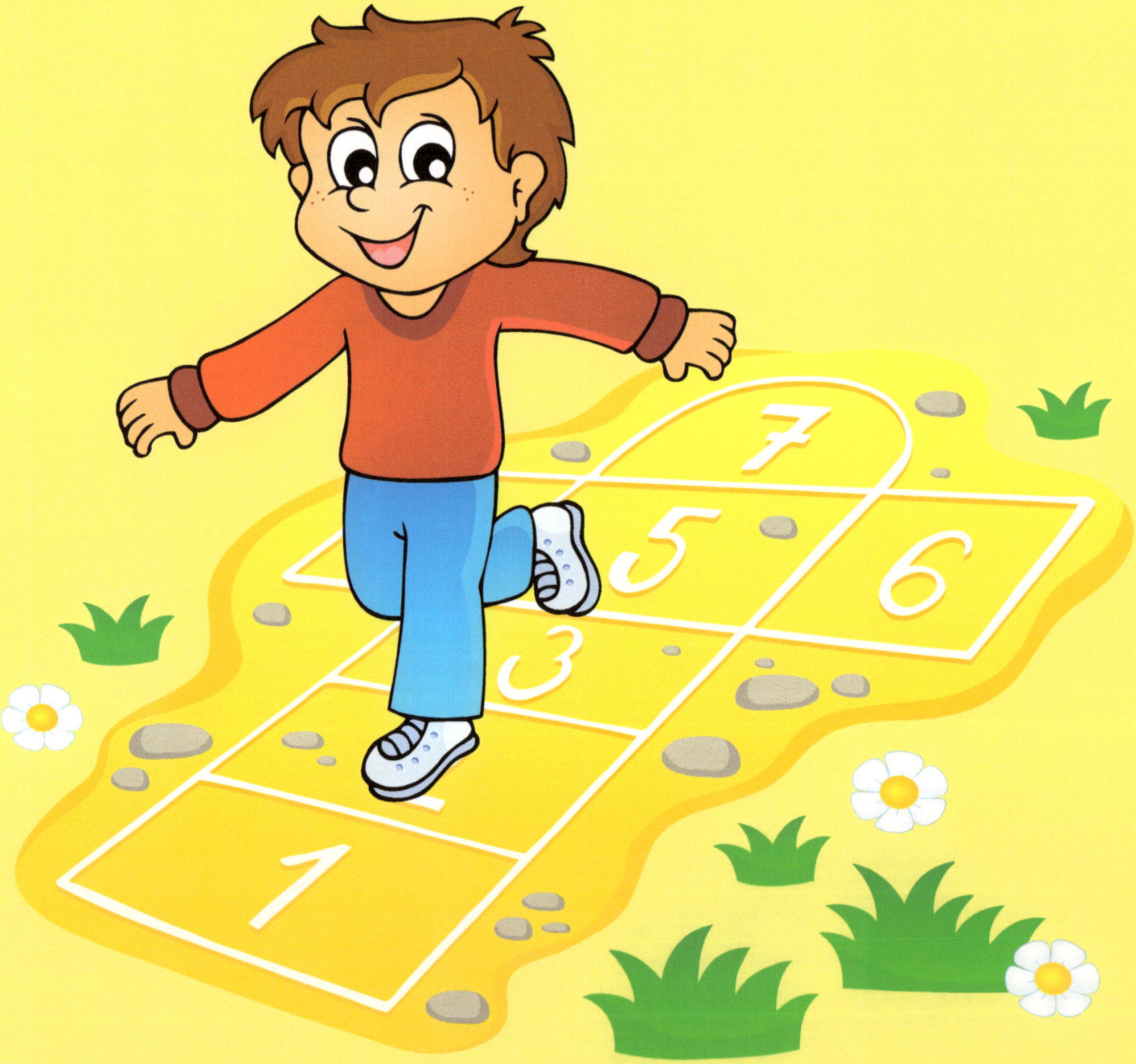

Play hopscotch with friends or all alone.
Toss a marker, bean-bag, coin, or stone.
From space to space I jump and hop,
grab the marker and will not stop!

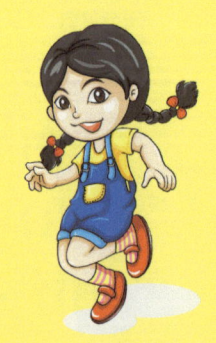

Ice Hockey

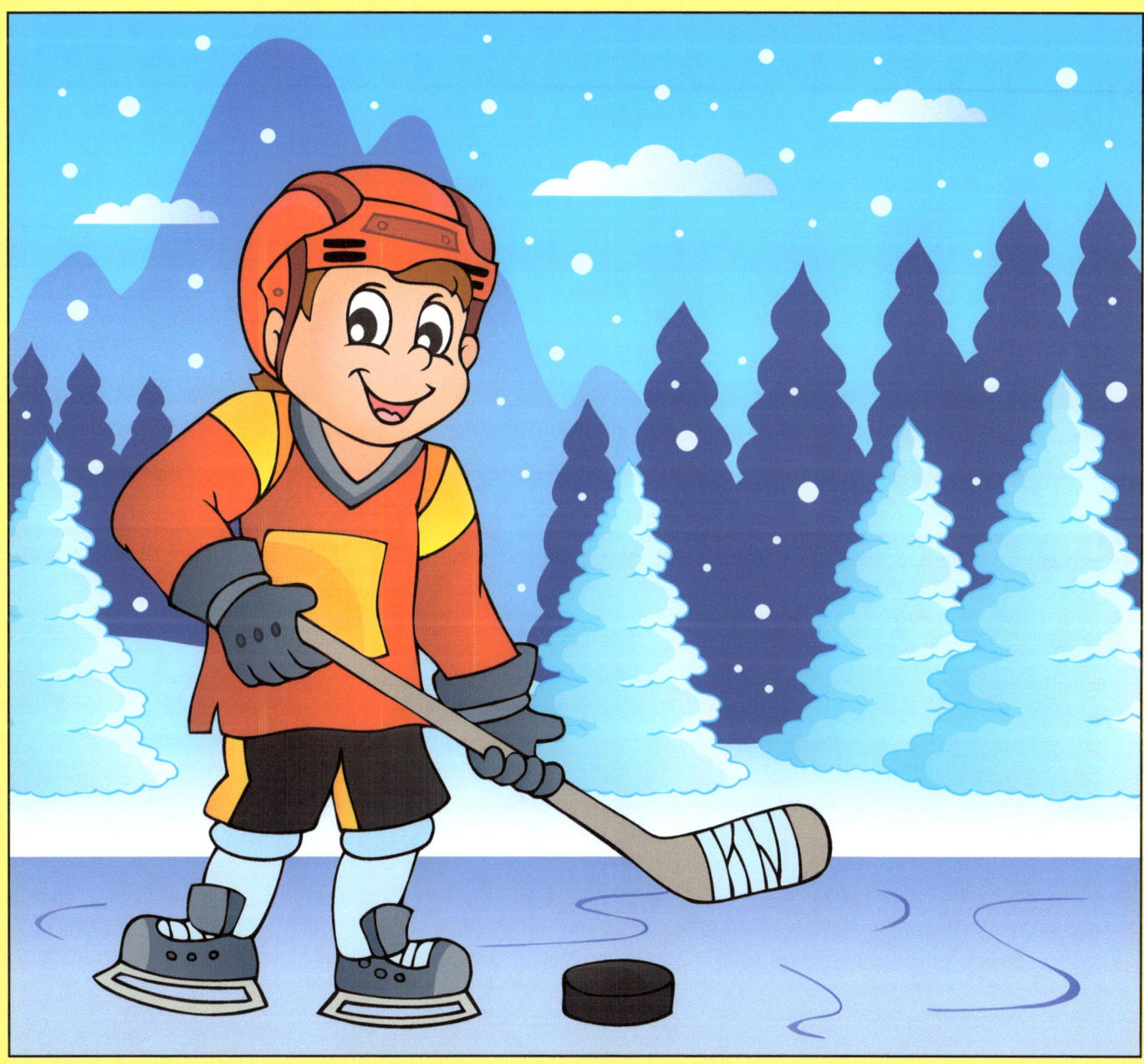

Hockey, a rough team sport, played on ice;
wear helmet and pads is my advice.
Skating, passing and shooting the puck with a stick,
flying toward the net, score a goal is the trick!

Jump

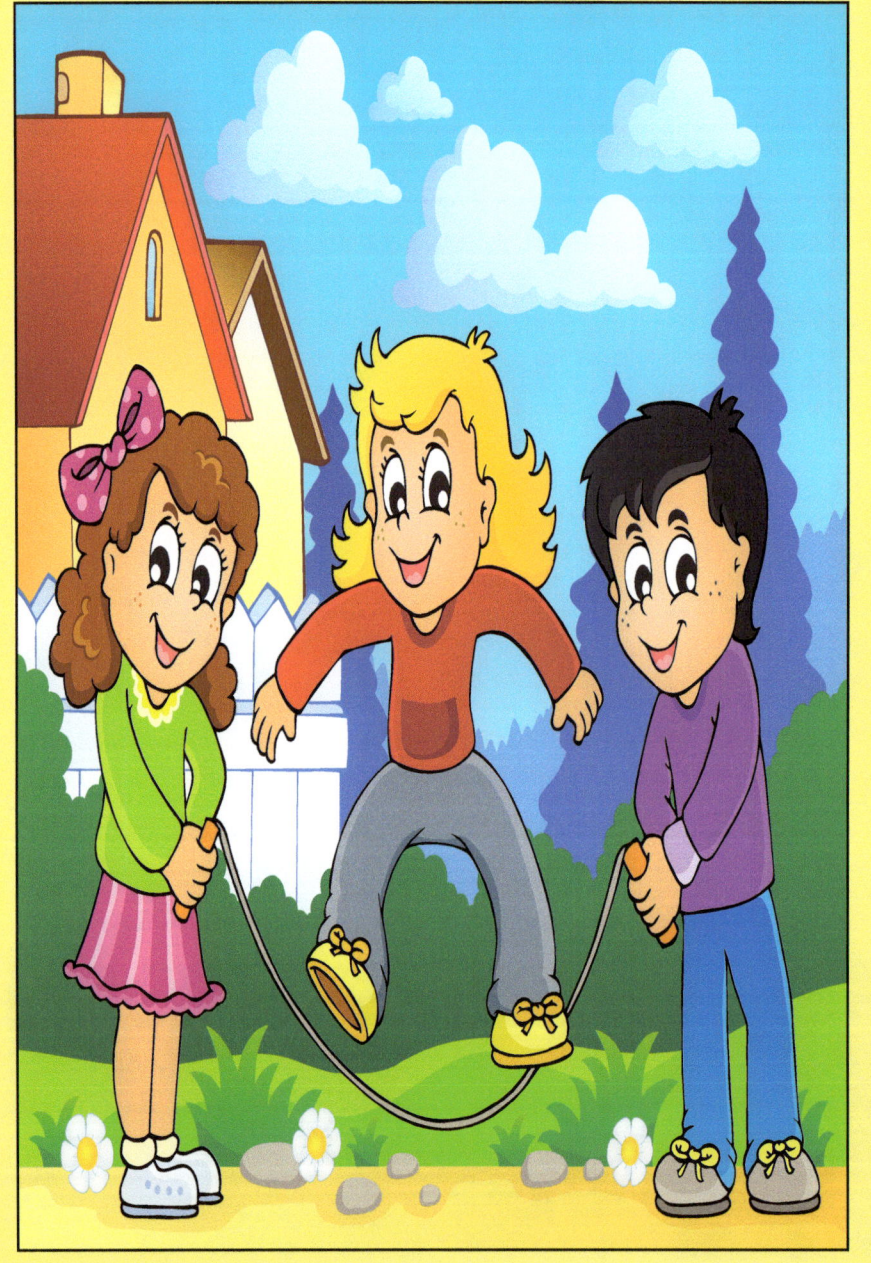
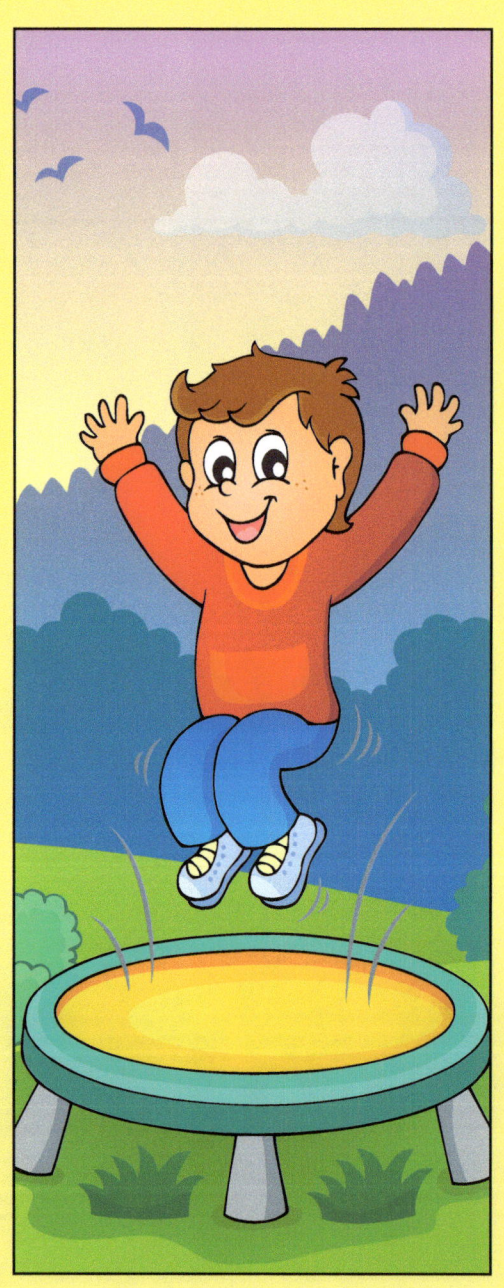

Jump, leap, or hop in the air,
with a rope or anywhere,
fast or slow, low or high,
with hands stretched toward the sky!

Kayak

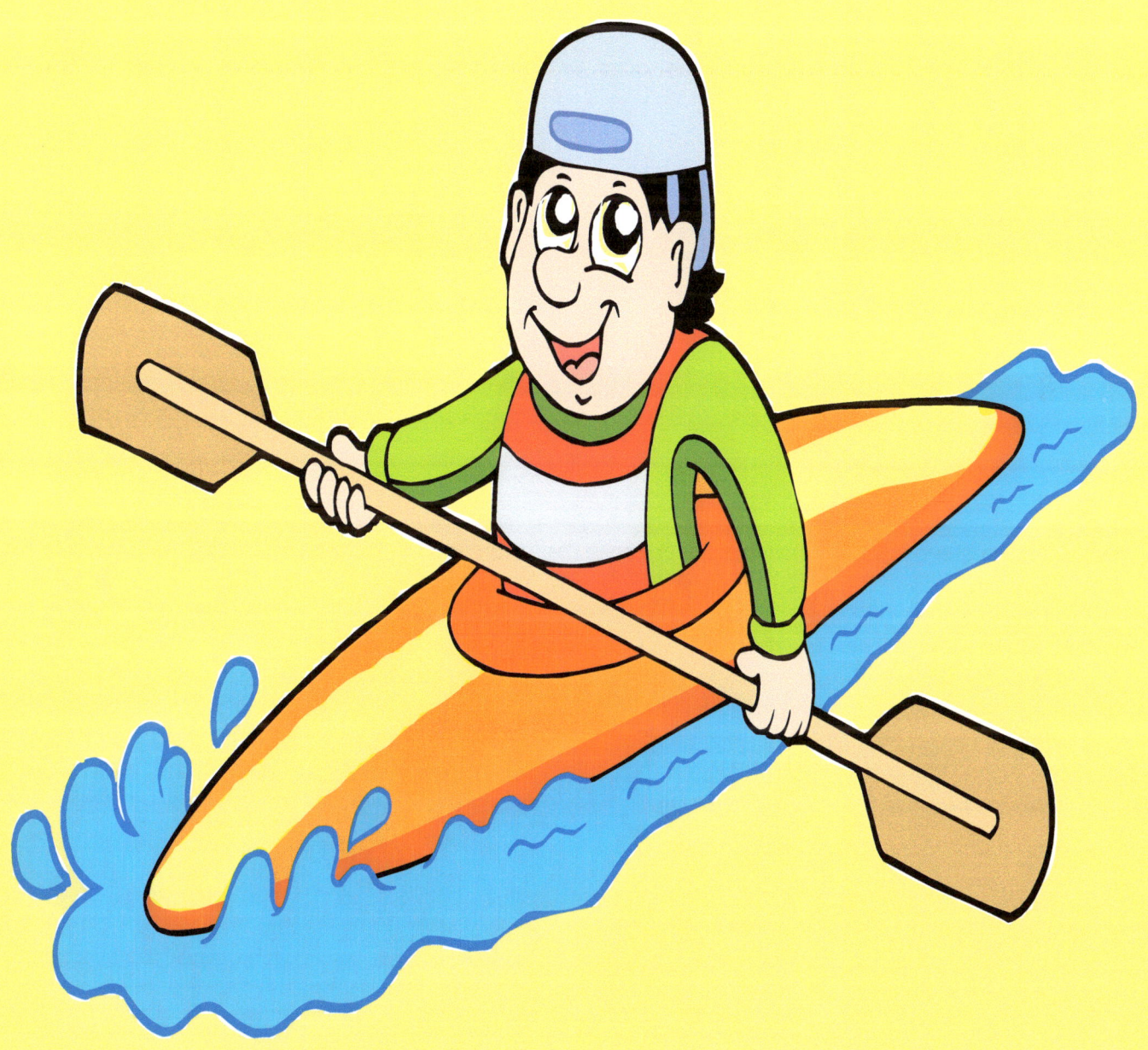

Low in the water a kayak will float.
I need a paddle to move this small boat.
I glide through water in a pond,
a lake, a river, and beyond.

LaCrosse

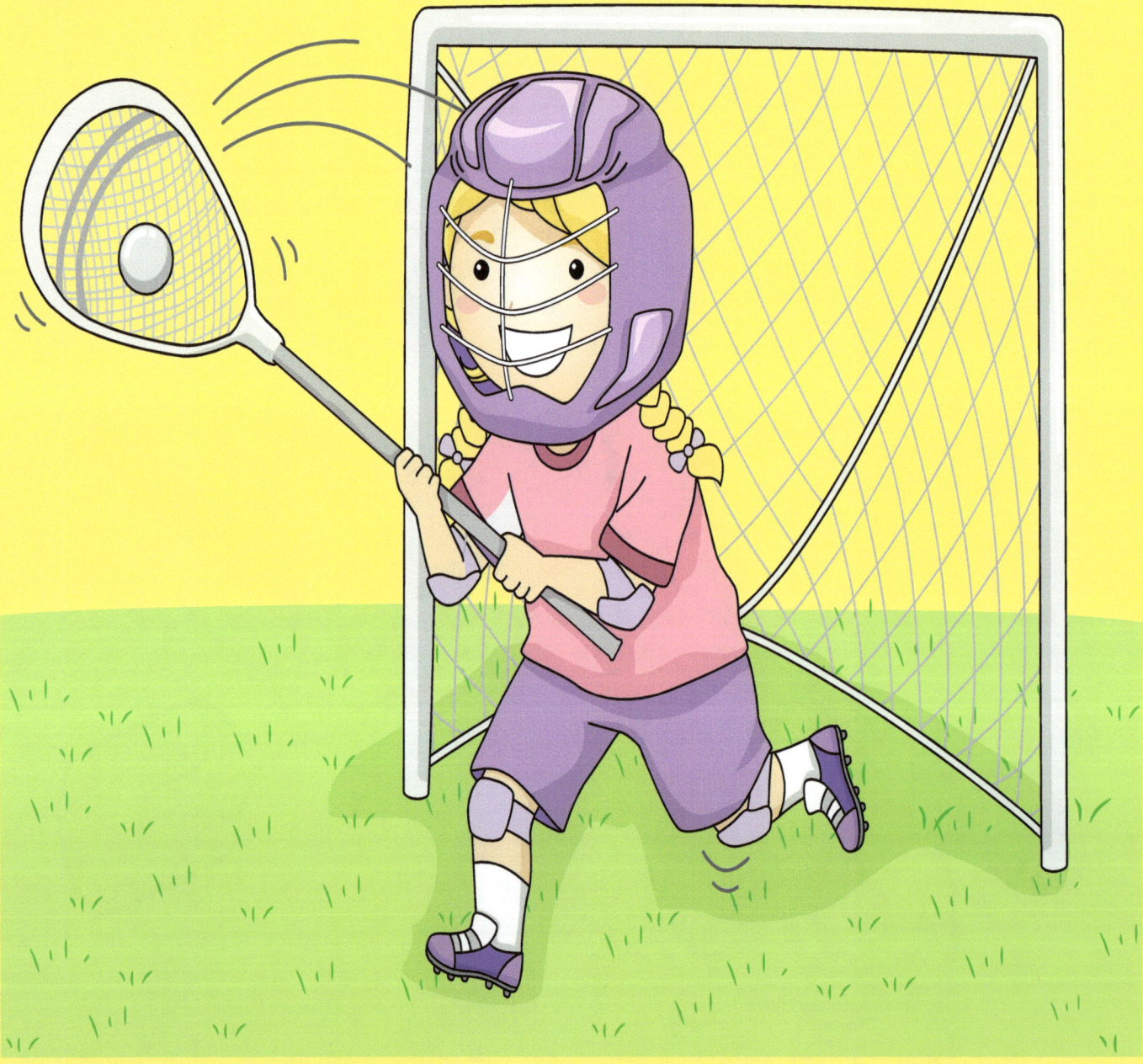

Lacrosse, a team sport, for those who like thrills,
with sticks and a ball, we practice our skills.
Catching, passing, shooting to score,
past the goalie my shot will soar!

Martial Arts

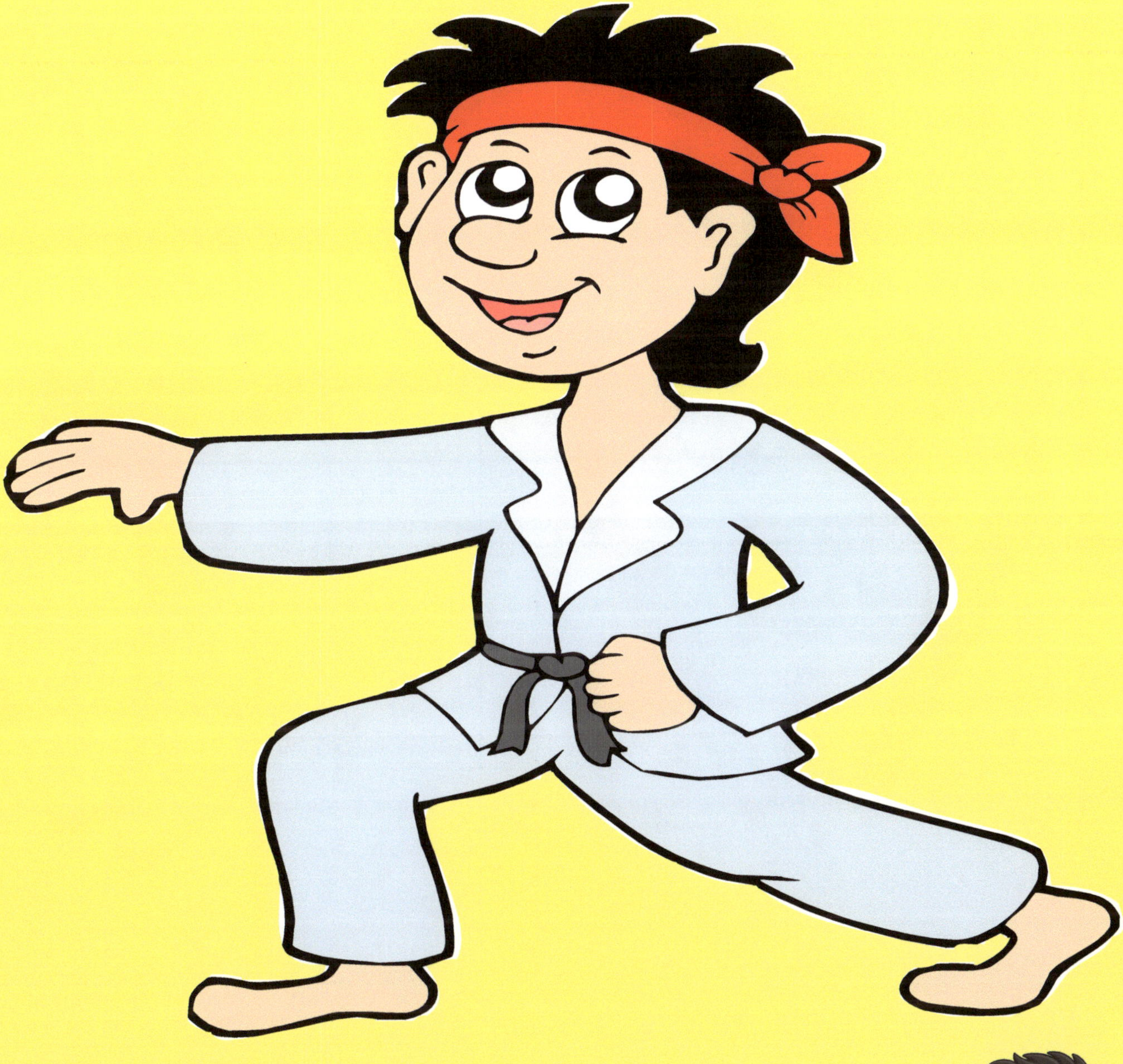

In martial arts, you learn strength and discipline before you're done. Punching, kicking, striking, and throwing are part of the fun.

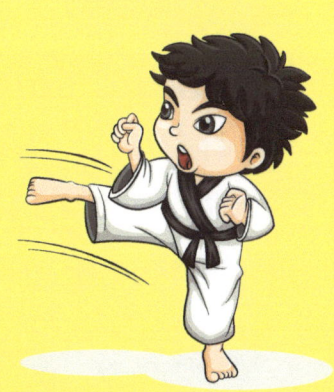

Nordic Skiing

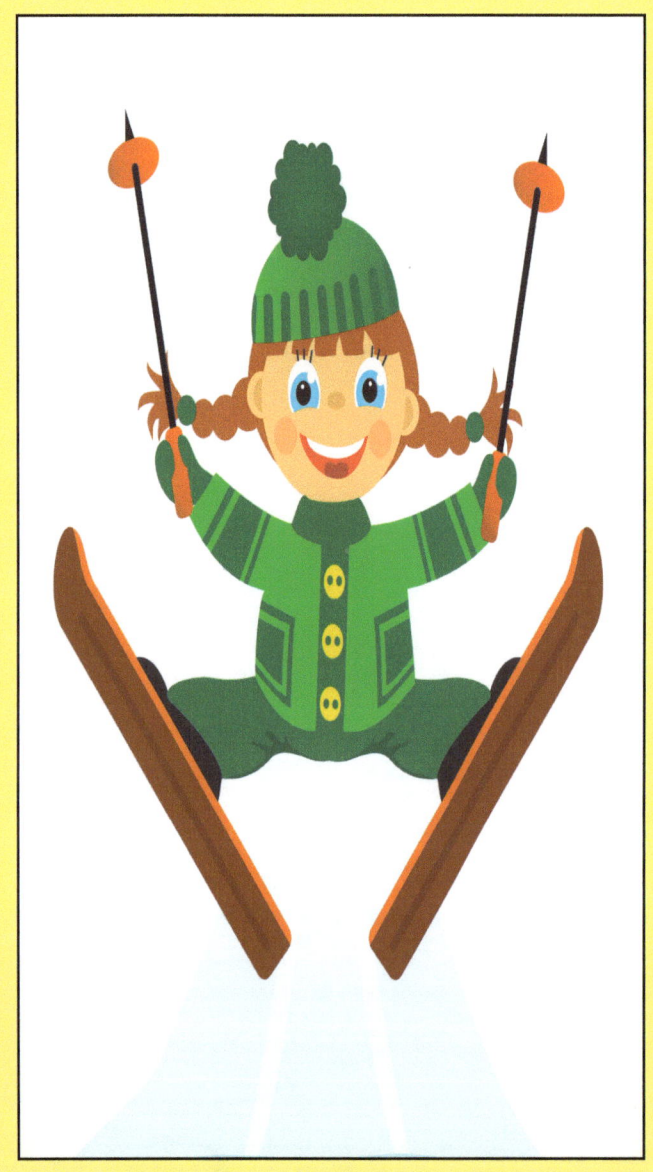
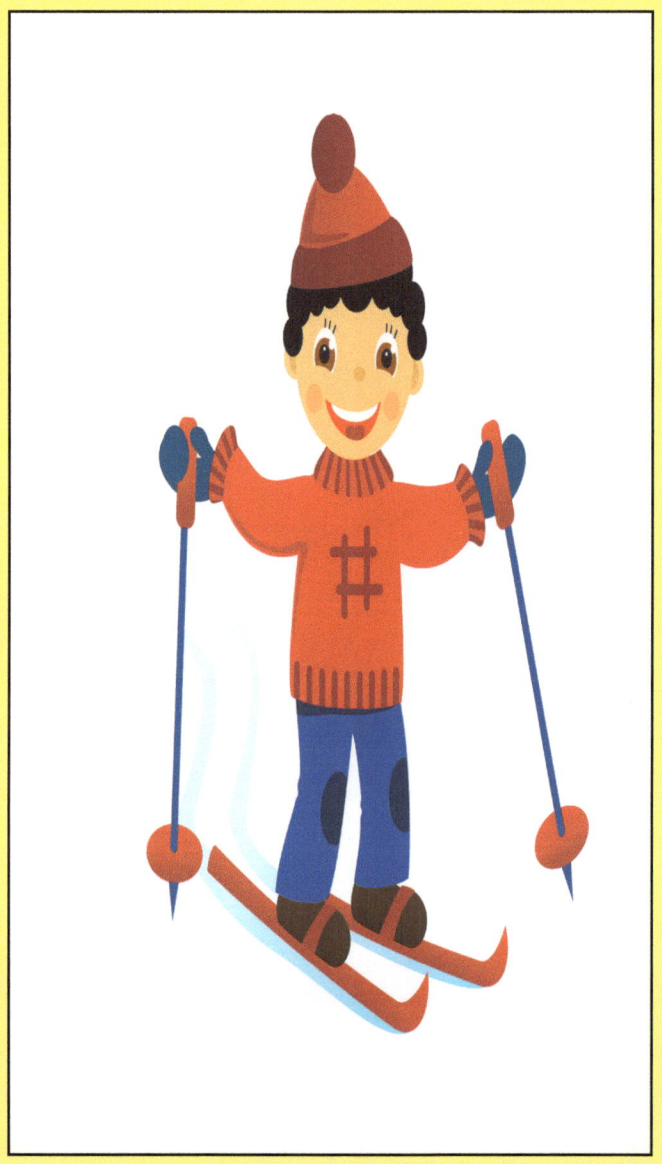

Nordic skiing is both ski jumping and cross country.
In both types, the boot heal is not attached to the ski.
Striding, sliding, I don't take a spill,
jumping and flying far down the hill.

Orienteering

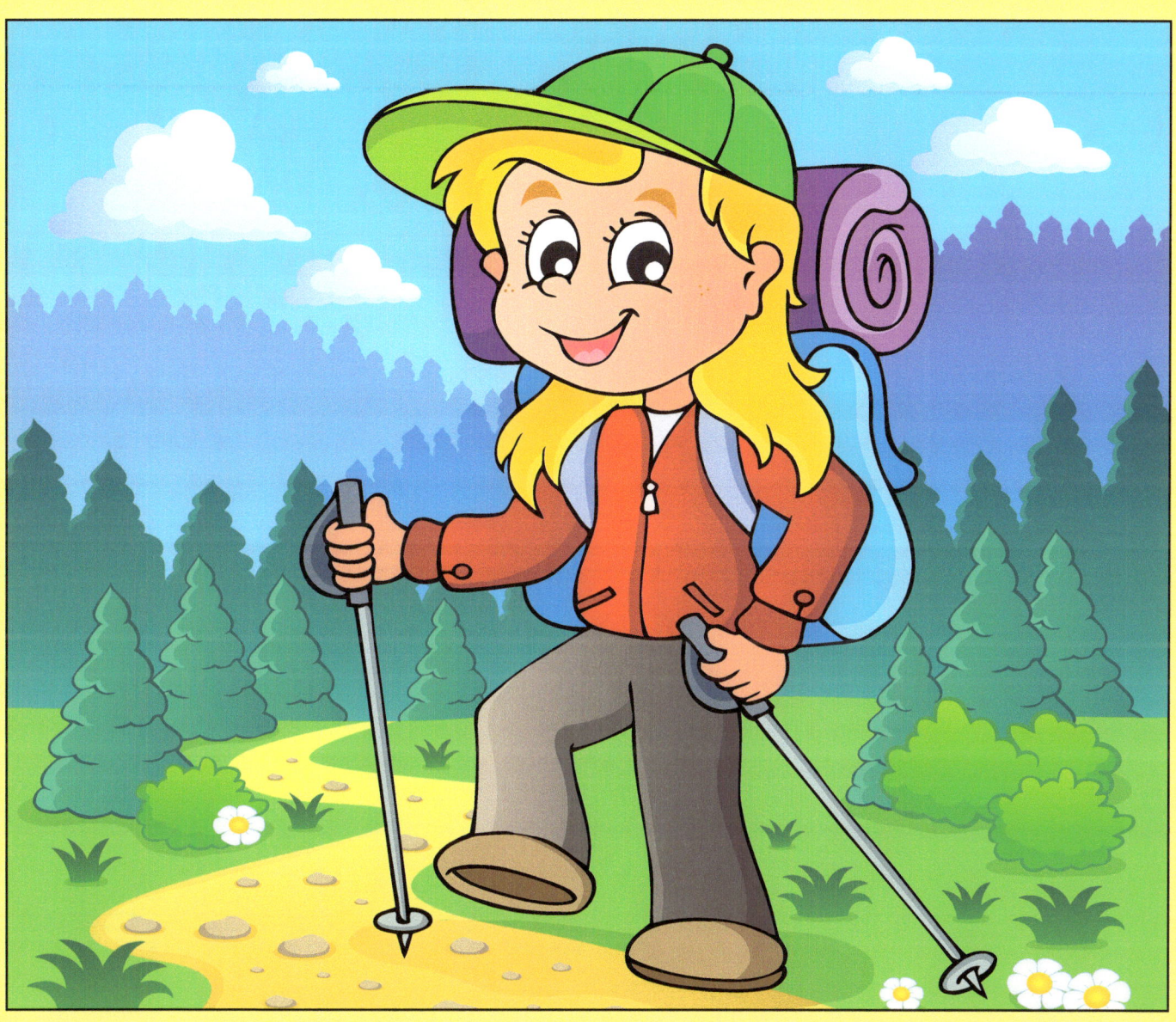

Orienteering from point-to-point is great!
With only map and compass, I navigate.

Ping Pong

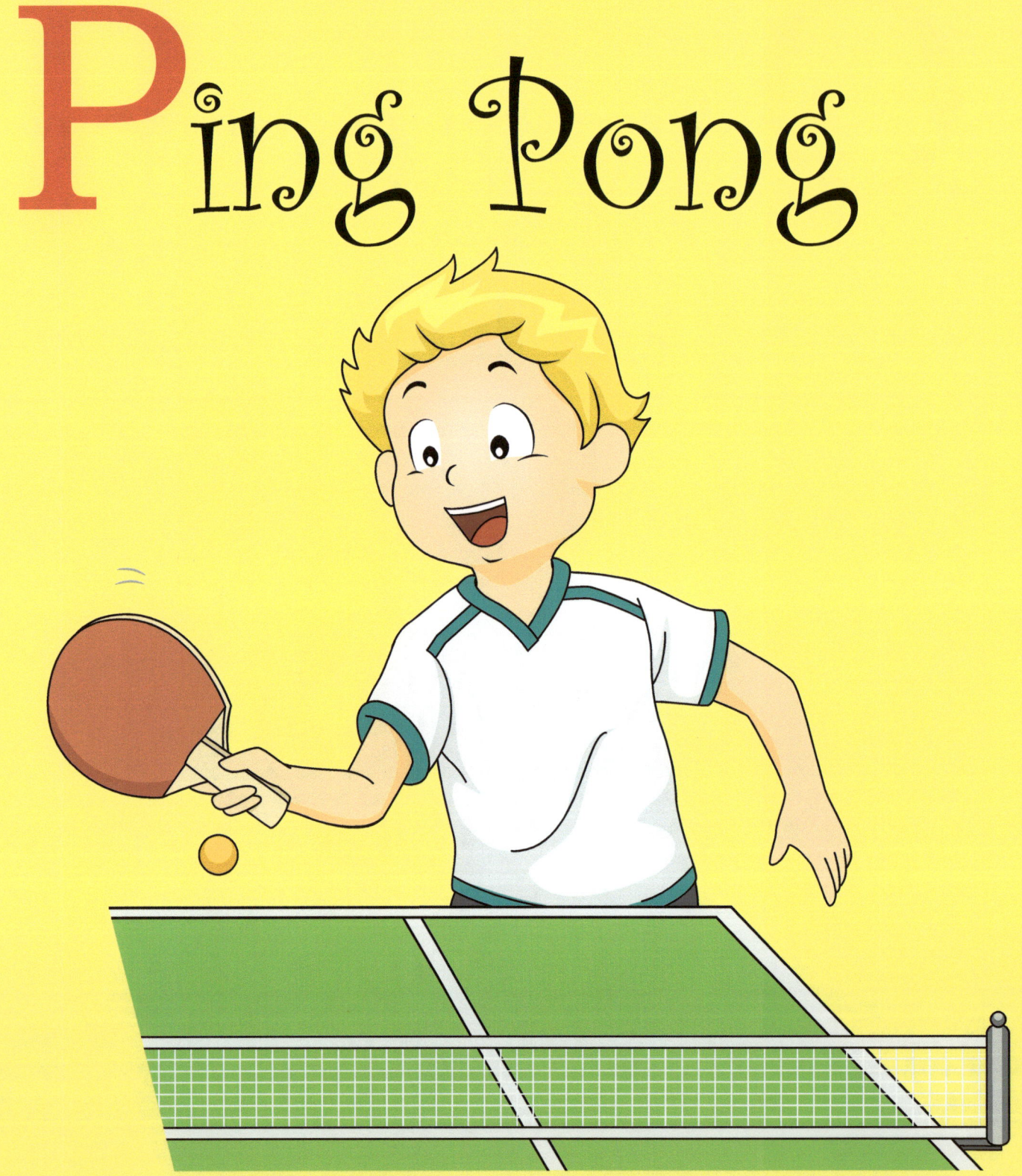

Played with paddle and ball on a hard table,
slamming it over the net if I'm able.
Ping pong or table tennis is played very fast.
Serving, spinning, and returning can be a blast!

Quick Step

Quick step dance tempo is very upbeat.
Dancers need to be light on their feet.
Hops, runs, and quick steps I take on with zeal.
Rotating briskly is part of the deal.

Riding

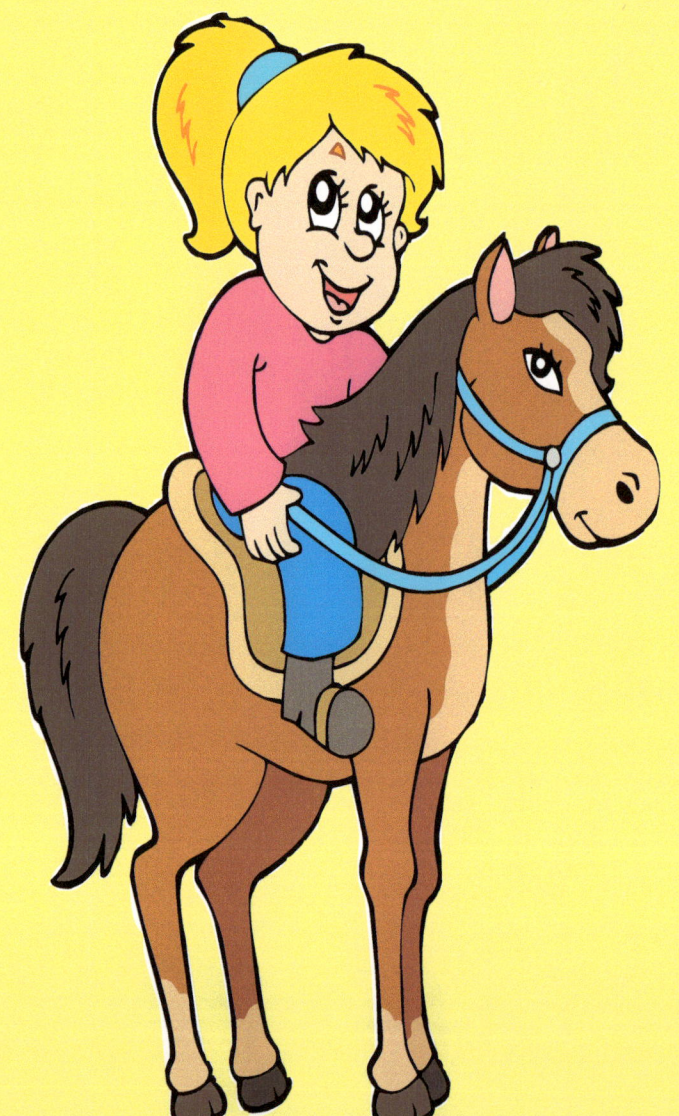

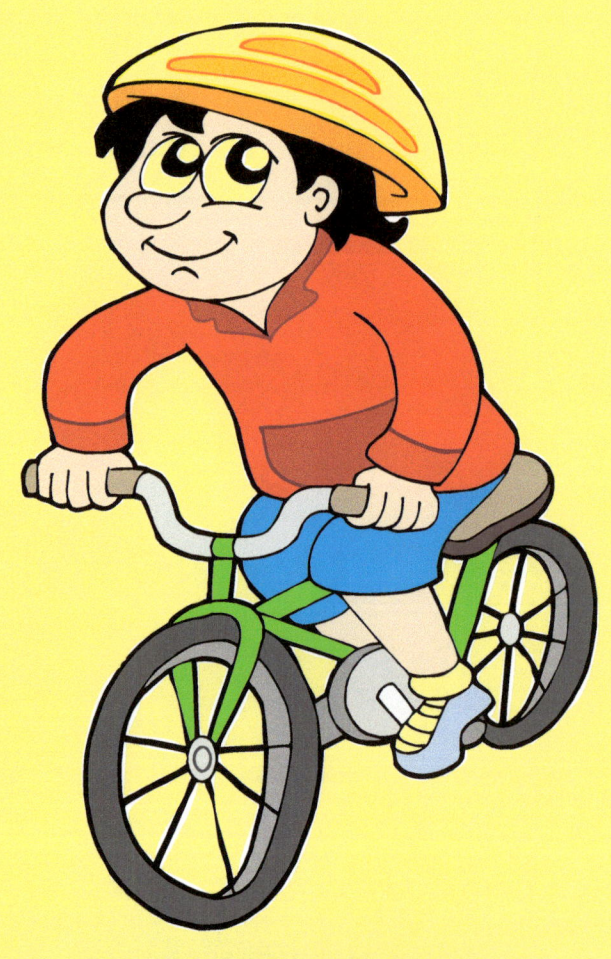

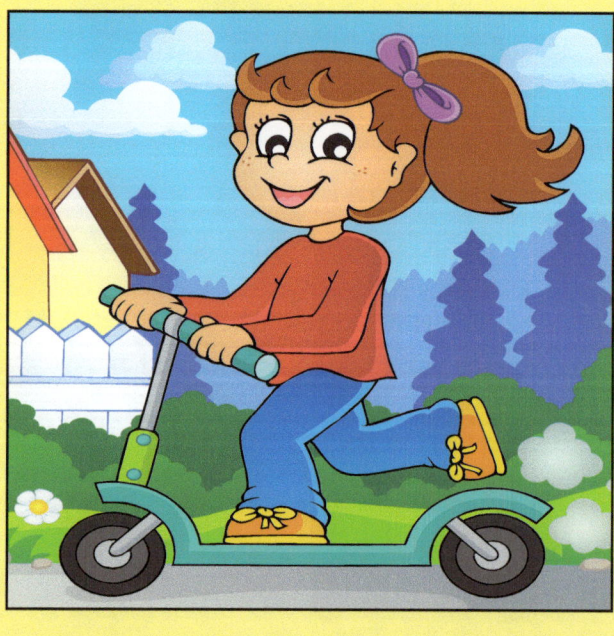

I ride a horse, a bike,
a scooter or a trike.
Riding is the way to go.
I can ride fast or slow!

Snow

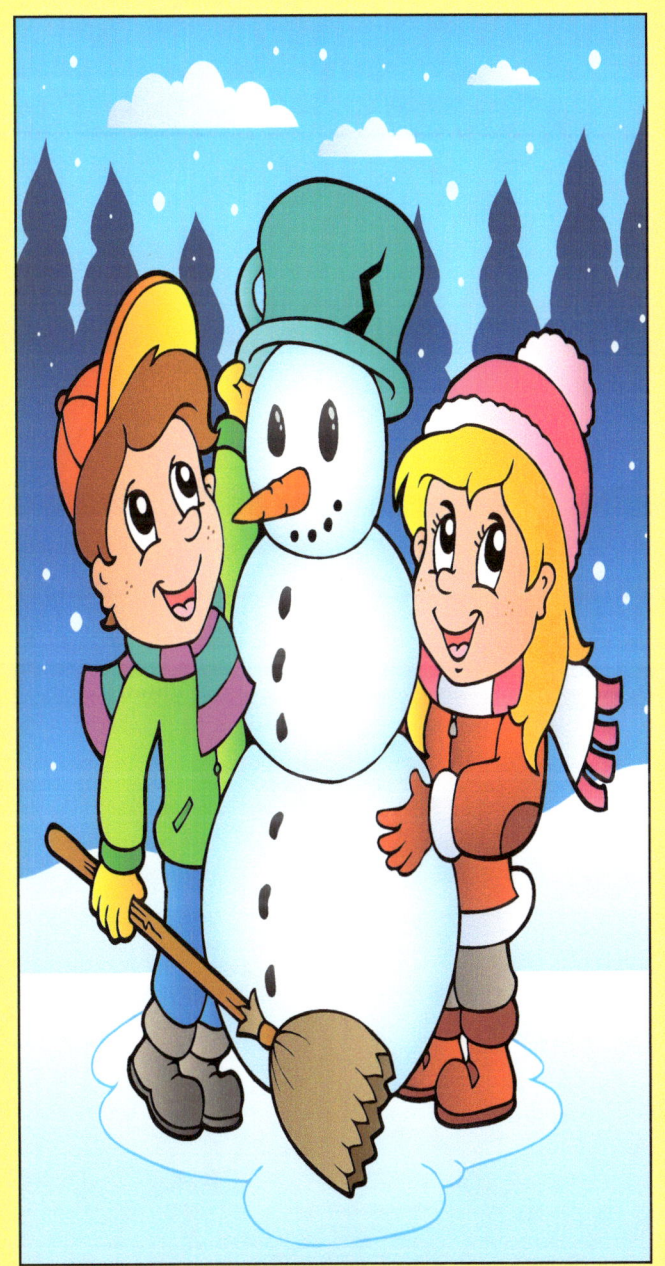

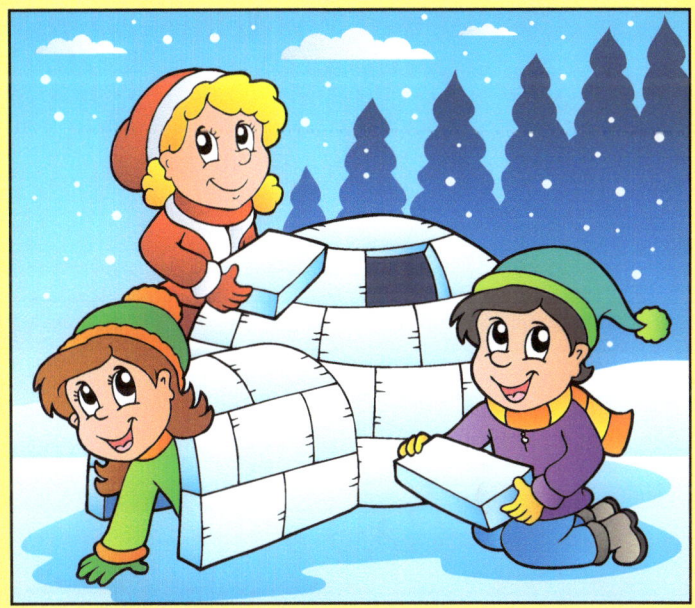

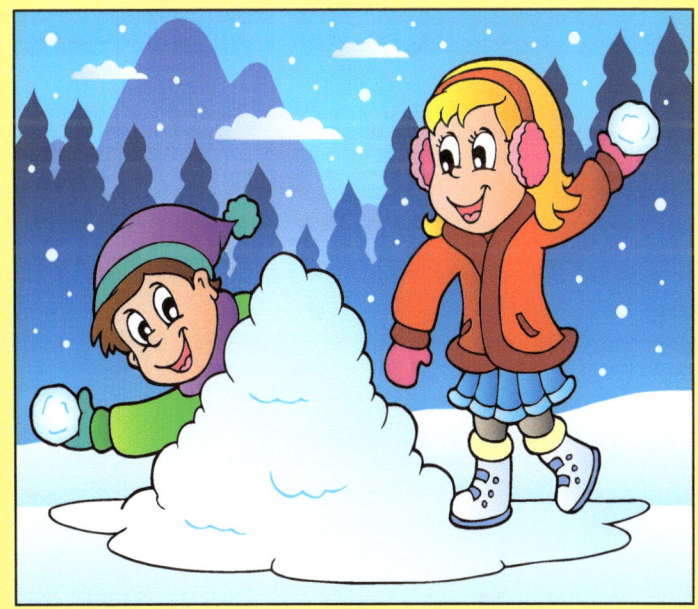

I love to play in the snow,
making snowballs I will throw.
Building a snowman and an igloo,
fun for all; it's a hullabaloo!

Tennis

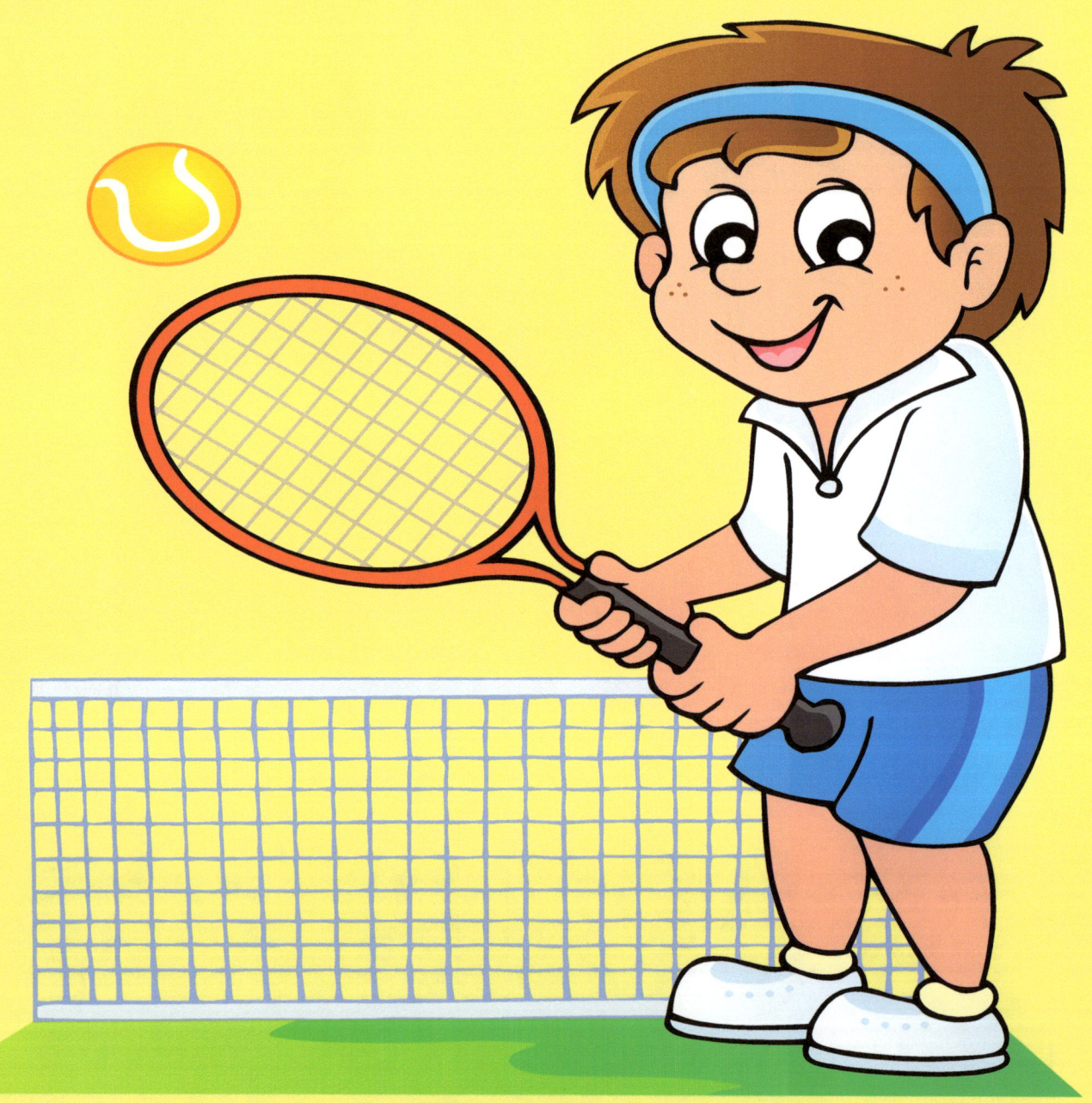

Tennis is my favorite sport.
I love to run around the court.
Forehand, backhand, rally 'til day is done,
volley, serve an ace, game, set, match, I won!

Unicycle

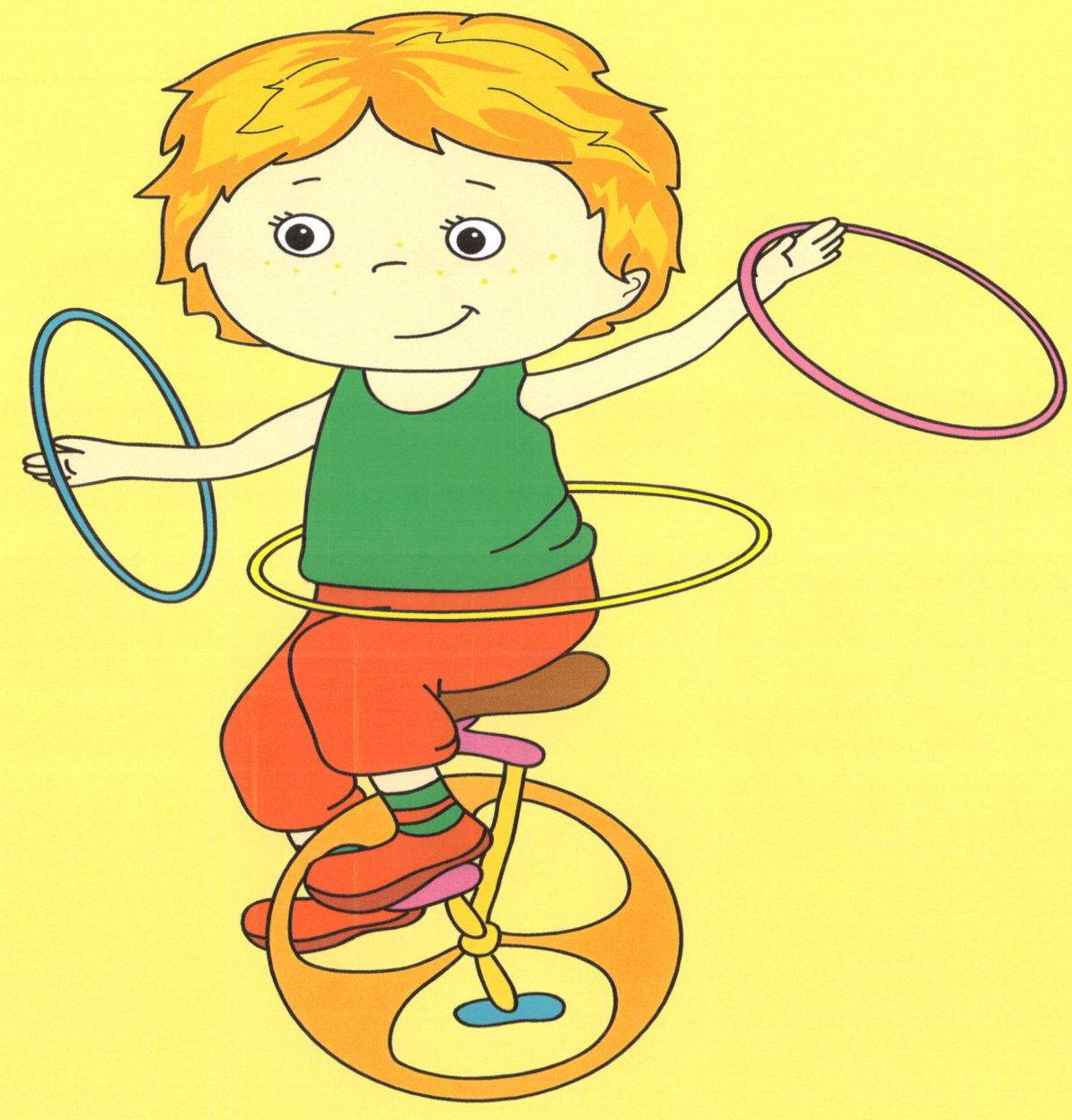

A unicycle has only one wheel.
Pedaling, balancing, make it ideal.
My hands are free to do other things.
I wave to my friends or twirl large rings!

Volleyball

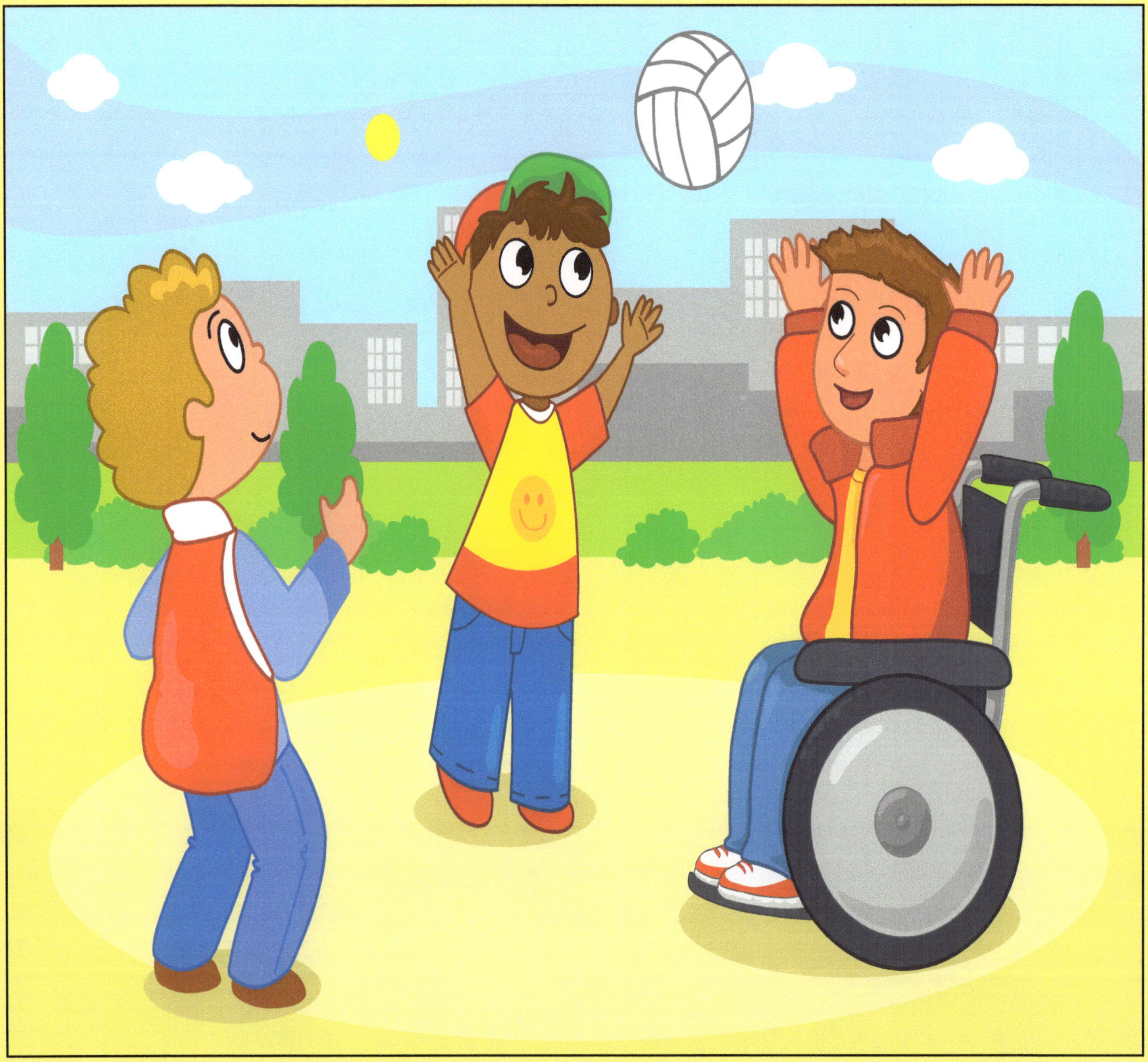

Serving, setting, attacking, bumping, passing, digging, blocking, and jumping; volleyball is an exciting game.
Hitting the ball is my claim to fame!

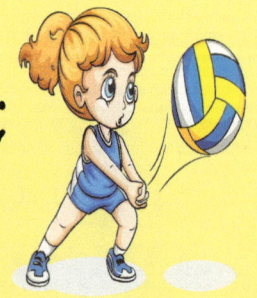

Water Fun

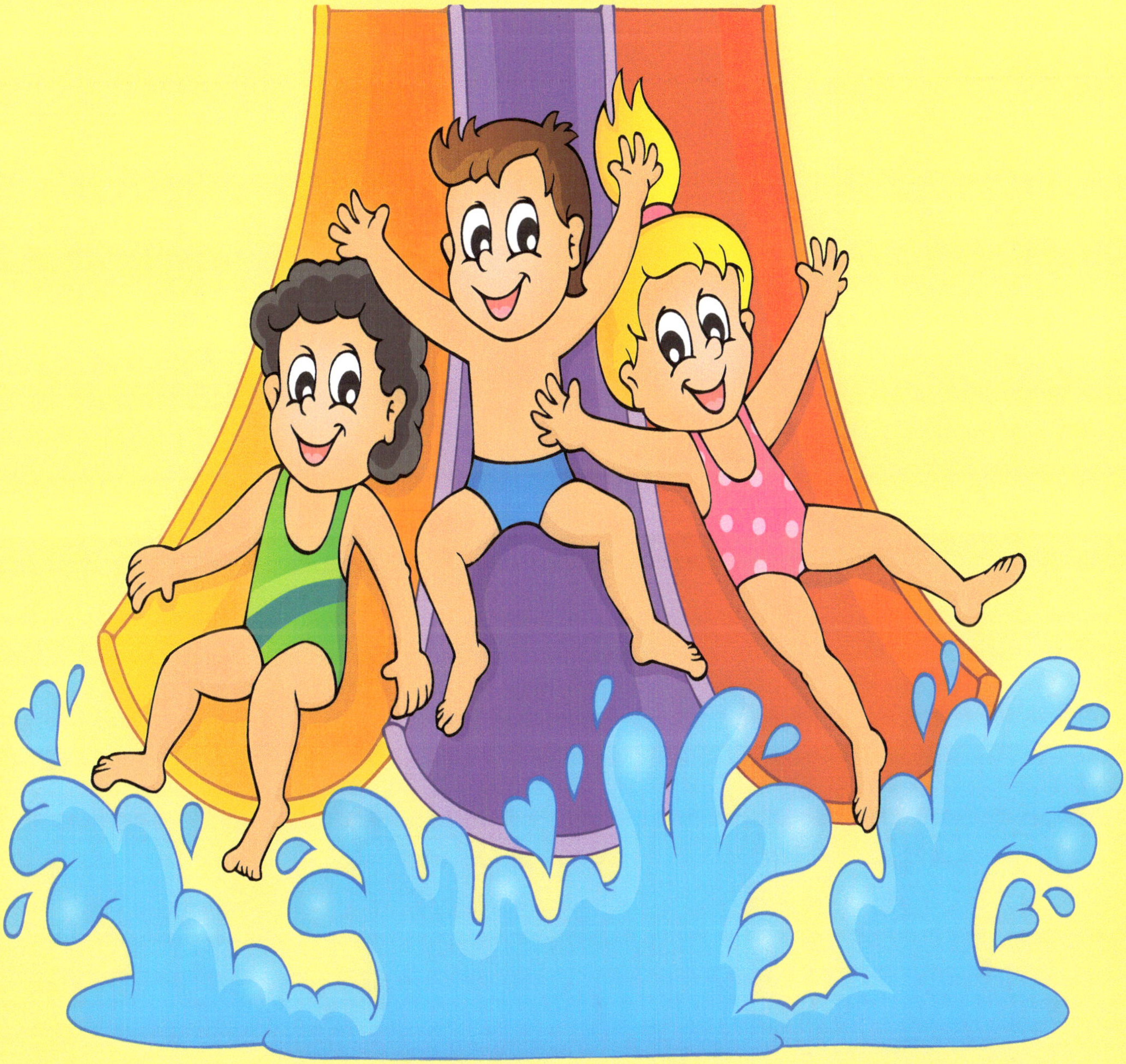

Water fun I recommend.
Be safe; always take a friend.
Sliding, diving, rafting, floating,
tubing, swimming, and row boating...

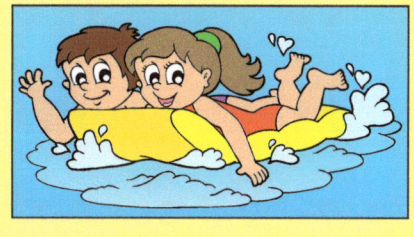

X-Games

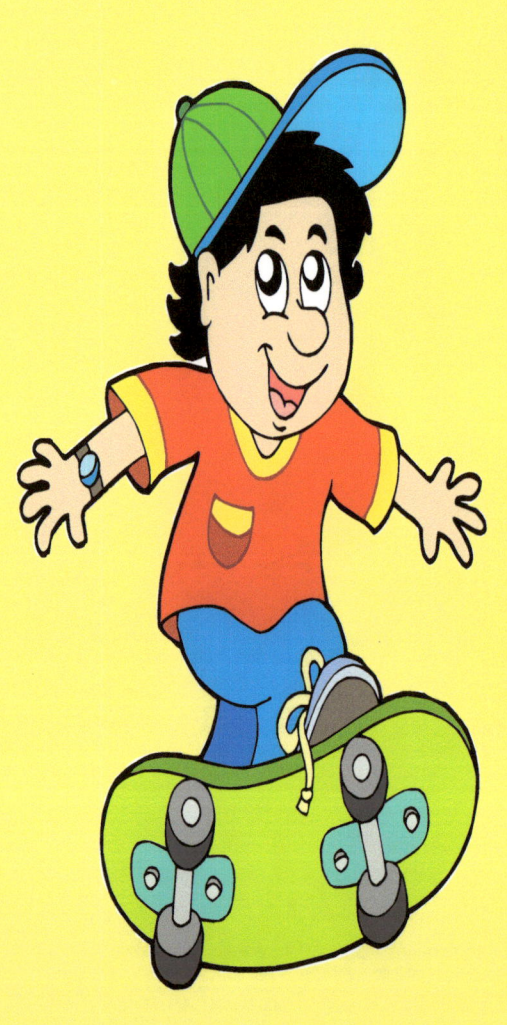

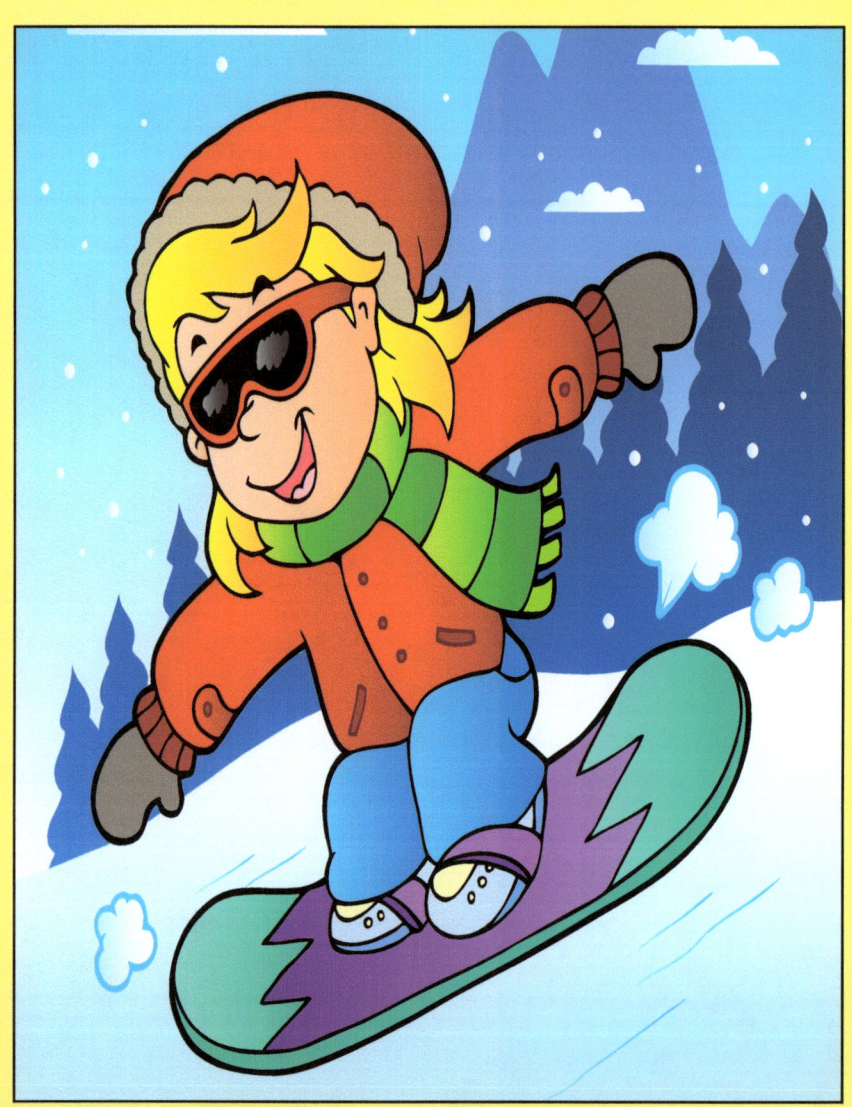

X-Game sports are always extreme,
faster, higher, never mainstream.
We compete in any season.
Pushing limits is our reason.
Snowboard, skateboard, surfboard and more;
I compete and want a high score!

Yoga

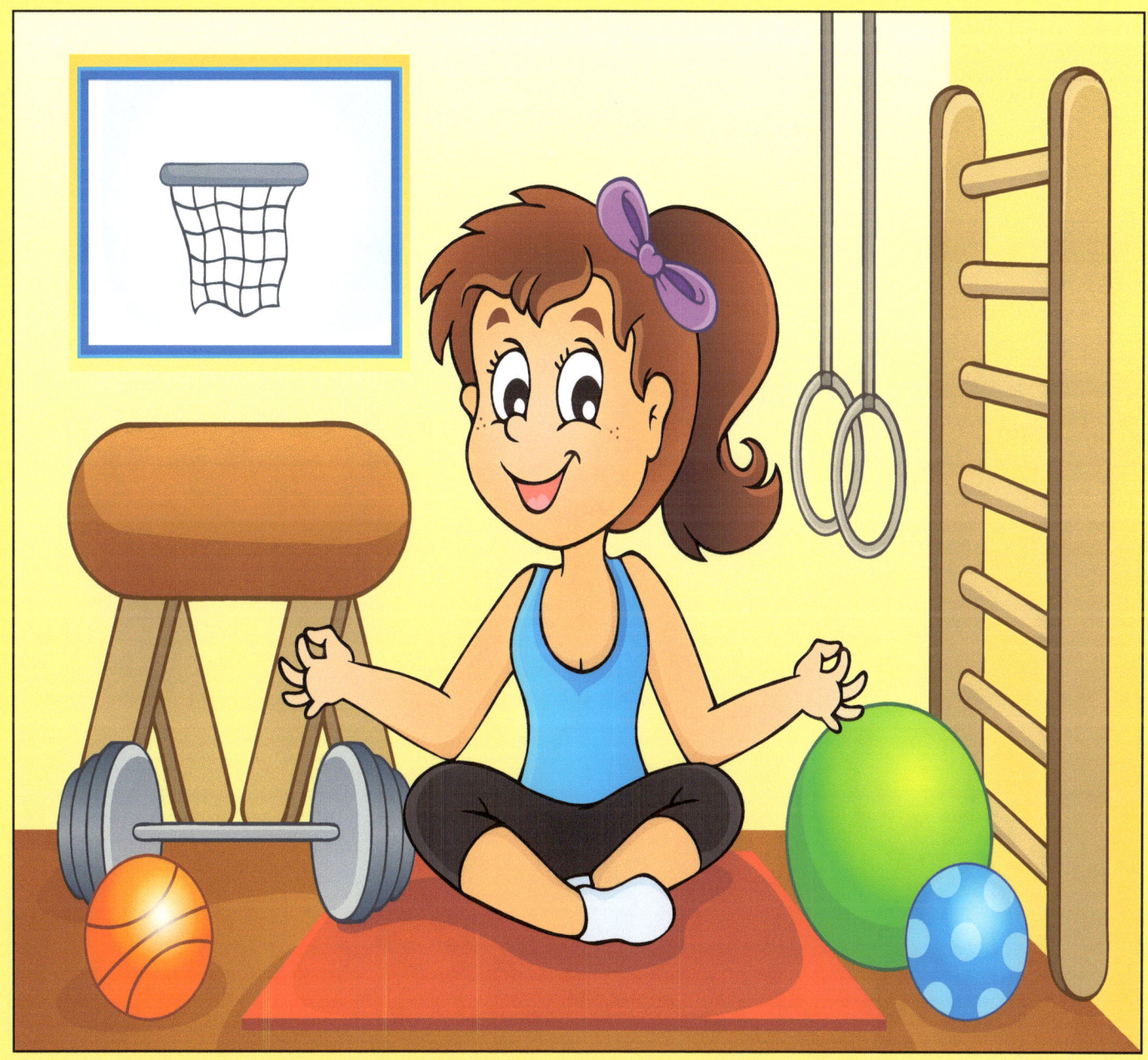

Flexibility is my goal.
A strength program I can control.
Postures or positions aid balance you'll find.
Yoga combines movements for body and mind.

Zip Line

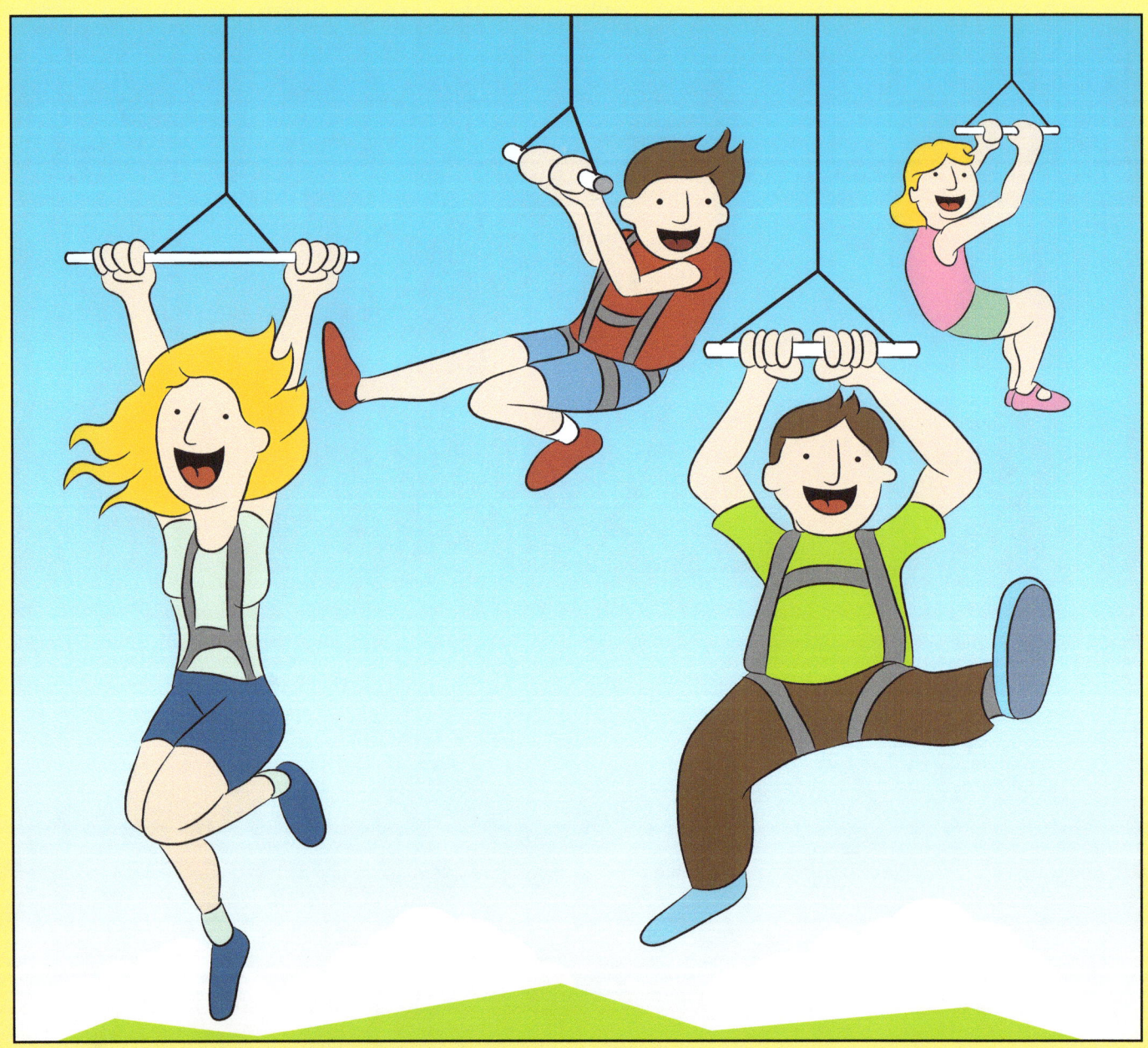

Zip lining fast or slow,
gravity makes you go.
Start up high and take flight;
I always hold on tight!

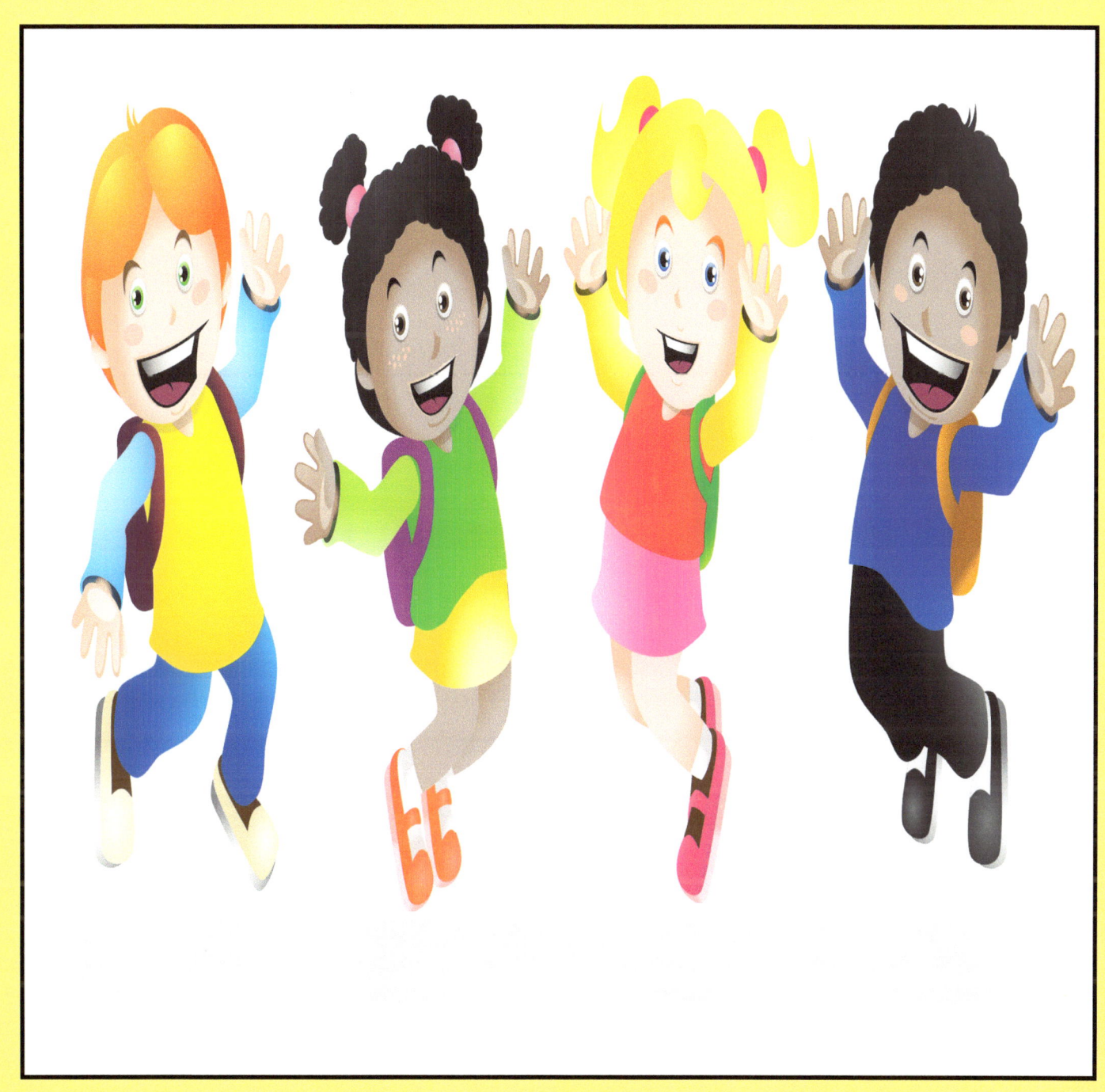

Now, the alphabet
is said and done.
Keep moving, because
fit kids have fun!

It's a simple rule, at home or at school, sixty minutes of play each and every day!

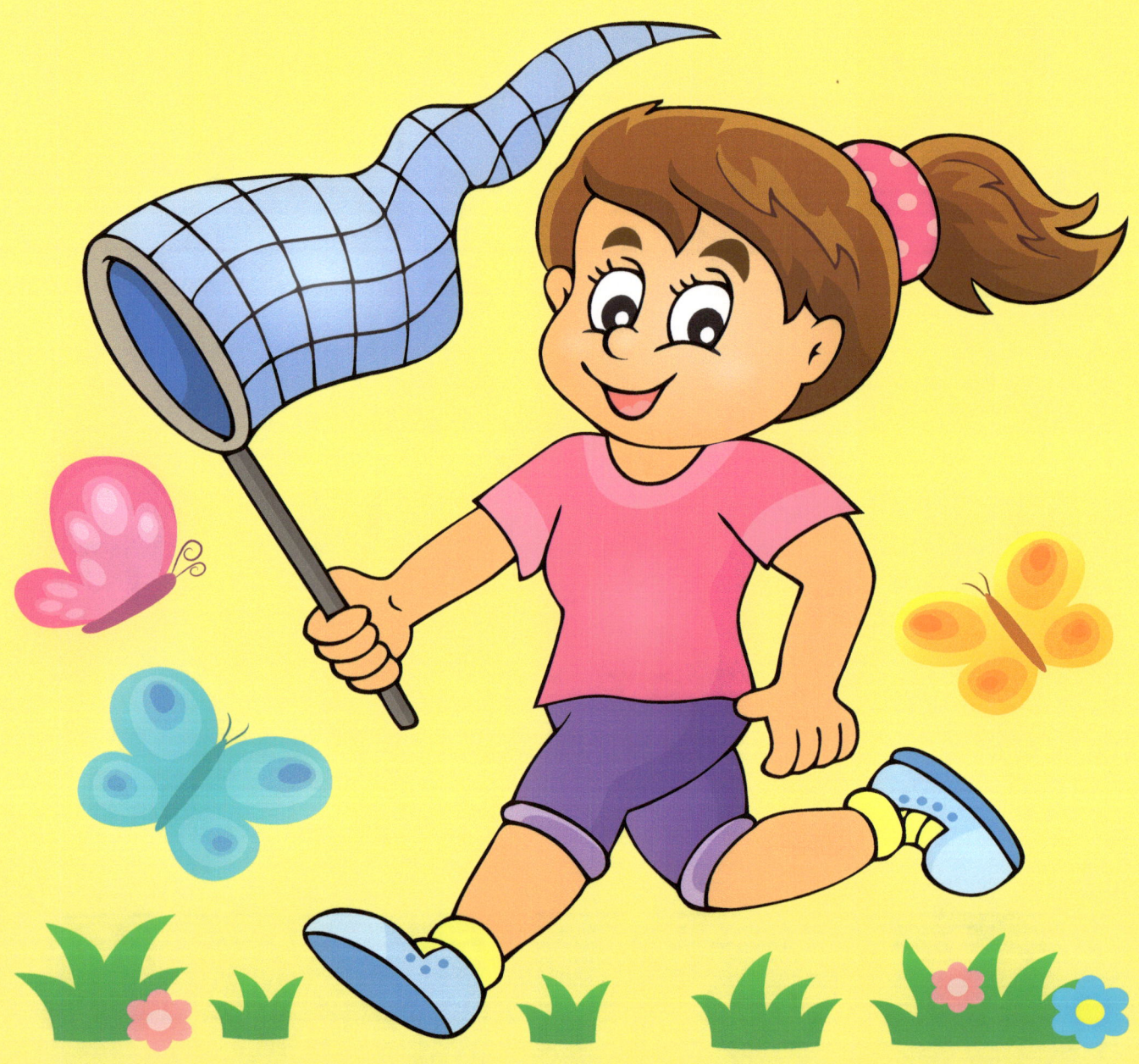

Adventure Learning Press
adventurelearningpress.com
adventurelearningpress@gmail.com

www.ingramcontent.com/pod-product-compliance
Lightning Source LLC
Chambersburg PA
CBHW060807290526

45792CB00005BA/1552